HW

Helping Children

Ros ary Wells grew up in Scotland and England, and settled in Africa
wh she married. On returning to England, she was widowed and left
w hree children. She is a former teacher, and still enjoys teaching
' workshops, but is now a freelance writer. She is the author of
g *Children Cope with Divorce*, *Making Friends with Your Stepchildren*
elping Children Cope with Change and Loss (all Sheldon Press).

Overcoming Common Problems Series

Selected titles

A full list of titles is available from Sheldon Press,
36 Causton Street, London SW1P 4ST and on our website at
www.sheldonpress.co.uk

Body Language: What You Need to Know
David Cohen

The Complete Carer's Guide
Bridget McCall

The Confidence Book
Gordon Lamont

Coping Successfully with Period Problems
Mary-Claire Mason

Coping with Age-related Memory Loss
Dr Tom Smith

Coping with Chemotherapy
Dr Terry Priestman

Coping with Compulsive Eating
Ruth Searle

Coping with Diverticulitis
Peter Cartwright

Coping with Family Stress
Dr Peter Cheevers

Coping with Hearing Loss
Christine Craggs-Hinton

Coping with Heartburn and Reflux
Dr Tom Smith

Coping with Macular Degeneration
Dr Patricia Gilbert

Coping with Radiotherapy
Dr Terry Priestman

Coping with Tinnitus
Christine Craggs-Hinton

The Depression Diet Book
Theresa Cheung

Depression: Healing Emotional Distress
Linda Hurcombe

Depressive Illness
Dr Tim Cantopher

The Fertility Handbook
Dr Philippa Kaye

Helping Children Cope with Anxiety
Jill Eckersley

How to Approach Death
Julia Tugendhat

How to Be a Healthy Weight
Philippa Pigache

How to Get the Best from Your Doctor
Dr Tom Smith

How to Make Life Happen
Gladeana McMahon

How to Talk to Your Child
Penny Oates

The IBS Healing Plan
Theresa Cheung

Living with Autism
Fiona Marshall

Living with Eczema
Jill Eckersley

Living with Heart Failure
Susan Elliot-Wright

Living with Loss and Grief
Julia Tugendhat

Living with a Seriously Ill Child
Dr Jan Aldridge

The Multiple Sclerosis Diet Book
Tessa Buckley

Overcoming Emotional Abuse
Susan Elliot-Wright

Overcoming Hurt
Dr Windy Dryden

The PMS Handbook
Theresa Cheung

Simplify Your Life
Naomi Saunders

Stress-related Illness
Dr Tim Cantopher

The Thinking Person's Guide to Happiness
Ruth Searle

The Traveller's Good Health Guide
Dr Ted Lankester

Treat Your Own Knees
Jim Johnson

Treating Arthritis – The Drug-Free Way
Margaret Hills

Overcoming Common Problems

Helping Children Cope with Grief

Facing a death in the family

Second edition

ROSEMARY WELLS

sheldon PRESS

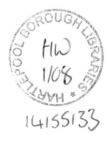

First published in Great Britain in 1988

Sheldon Press
36 Causton Street
London SW1P 4ST

Reprinted 7 times
Second edition published 2007

The author and publisher have made every effort to ensure that the
external website and email addresses included in this book are correct and
up to date at the time of going to press. The author and publisher are not
responsible for the content, quality or continuing accessibility of the sites.

British Library Cataloguing-in-Publication Data
A catalogue record for this book is available from the British Library

ISBN 978-1-84709-022-5

1 3 5 7 9 10 8 6 4 2

Typeset by Fakenham Photosetting Ltd, Fakenham, Norfolk
Printed in Great Britain by Ashford Colour Press

Produced on paper from sustainable forests

Overcoming Common Problems

Helping Children Cope with Grief

Facing a death in the family

Second edition

ROSEMARY WELLS

sheldon**PRESS**

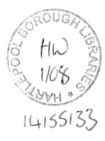

First published in Great Britain in 1988

Sheldon Press
36 Causton Street
London SW1P 4ST

Reprinted 7 times
Second edition published 2007

The author and publisher have made every effort to ensure that the
external website and email addresses included in this book are correct and
up to date at the time of going to press. The author and publisher are not
responsible for the content, quality or continuing accessibility of the sites.

British Library Cataloguing-in-Publication Data
A catalogue record for this book is available from the British Library

ISBN 978-1-84709-022-5

1 3 5 7 9 10 8 6 4 2

Typeset by Fakenham Photosetting Ltd, Fakenham, Norfolk
Printed in Great Britain by Ashford Colour Press

Produced on paper from sustainable forests

Contents

Acknowledgements

I should like to express my sincere thanks to all the people who helped and encouraged me while writing this book: the families who so willingly shared their memories and experiences; the many teachers, doctors, consultants in child psychiatry, mental handicap, and paediatrics; ministers of religion, nurses, social workers, counsellors, and other experts in their own fields who have given generously of their time and advice; senior officers and students in the police, ambulance, and other public services.

My thanks also to those who made me so welcome in their caring organizations: Cruse Bereavement Care, The Compassionate Friends, the Lisa Sainsbury Foundation, the National Children's Home, the Westminster Pastoral Foundation, St Christopher's Hospice, Princess Alice Hospice, Helen House, the Royal College of Nursing, Macmillan Home Care Service.

I am gratefully indebted to the experts whose papers, lectures, tapes and videos were made freely available to me, notably: Dr Janet Goodall, Dr Dora Black, Dr Richard Lansdown, Professor Joan Bicknell, Mrs Jane Davies, the Revd Canon Michael Kitchener.

Finally, to all who have gi n up so much time to talk with me, to discuss viewpoints anc ve advice: Mrs Jane Barry, Ariel Bruce, Dr Hamish Cameron, ı Amar Chhatwall, Mrs Penny Crawley, Mother Frances Dominica, Elizabeth Earnshaw-Smith, Lynn Franchino, Barbara Greenall, Dr Sheila Hollins, the Revd A. Glyn Jones, Mrs Benita Kyle, Father Tom McKenna, Rabbi Julia Neuberger, Mrs Margaret Nuttall, Mrs P. M. Turley, Mrs Jill Waller.

I owe so much to them all – not least to Barbara Pentreath who supported me from the start, and to both Anne-Marie

Edwards and Darley Anderson who gave me the faith to begin.

I should also like to thank all those, especially the young families, who helped with this new edition, including Barbara Bowen, John Morris and Barbara Ward.

Preface

The dictionary defines grief as 'deep or violent sorrow'. Grief sounds such a grown-up word and yet emotional bereavement in a child goes as deep as it does for an adult. Its effects are devastating, and may persist for years.

'I felt the bottom of my world falling out,' said Emily, who had to face her father's death when she was only 6 years old, leaving her with a grief-stricken mother unable to cope, and a resentful older sister. The safe family life she knew vanished overnight.

Ernest H. Shepard, whose unforgettable drawings brought A. A. Milne's *Winnie the Pooh* to life, wrote in his memoirs of his mother's early death, which 'cut short our happy family life ... It was years before the cloud seemed to lift and the natural buoyancy and happiness of youth revived itself in me.'

Every day, there are children who suffer the death of someone close to them. In England and Wales alone in one day 40 children under 16 will lose a mother or father.

In the last two or three decades, attitudes to death, bereavement and grieving have altered, and many organizations now exist that are able to help families faced with tragic situations (see Useful addresses, page 113). If your own children, or others in your care, are suffering from such grief, you may find in this book stories which help you learn how other families have survived. Bereavement can be isolating, but reading of experiences – however different from your own – may reveal emotions that make you think, 'Yes, that's how it feels!'

Rosemary Wells

1

Grief in childhood

There is a tendency to describe bereaved children, as well as children of divorced couples, as members of 'one-parent families'. The majority may be those from divided homes, and such children suffer deeply; their sense of loss must never be underestimated. But children who have suffered their loss through the death of a parent have special problems and needs that must be acknowledged and tackled if they are not to suffer unduly, perhaps even into adulthood. This includes even the youngest members of the family – they must never be forgotten.

Children's perception of death

Many studies have been carried out to determine children's perception of death. Analytical tables can appear very clinical (I have not reproduced any here for that reason) but are undertaken for and by the many professionals involved in the care of dying children and their siblings. They know that to be able to communicate with these children is vital, and they can only do so effectively if they can 'tune in' to the correct level of understanding each child has reached.

Helpful as these are, the professionals themselves are the first to emphasize that they can only be taken as guidelines. In order to help a particular child we have to watch for his or her individual perceptions. I've heard more than one expert say that, even after years of working among bereaved children, they are 'constantly surprised by how much small children *do* understand'.

Signs of sorrow even in babies of, say, 6 to 18 months can be seen. Once they can recognize a person, that person's absence becomes a huge loss. More than usual crying, shaking the bars of a cot – even the banging of a little head against them – all express strong emotions that will take time to comfort with extra love and attention.

From 2 to 5 years, a child learns trust – Mummy goes out, but she returns. Somewhere in those years he hears death mentioned – sees a dead bird or is read a sad fairy tale, and understands dead as being 'not alive'. Again, concepts will vary. A 4-year-old talking of his hamster said, 'He's dead, we buried him,' but a week later was seen digging in the garden 'to see if he's woken up yet'.

From 5 to 8 years, there is a gradual awareness of death as irrevocable. This may cause guilt feelings – a child may think his dad's death is a punishment for his naughty behaviour. Alternatively, a child can *become* naughty, fool about, pretend not to care. This may well be denial: Daddy *can't* be dead!

The realization that they too will die, and the difficult grasp of abstract concepts, does not come overnight. It is a gradual awareness, accelerated by a child's own experiences. She may be only 5 years old, but through family tragedy, or living in a country at war, or because of a highly developed intelligence, she may well hold concepts of death more usual in an 8-year-old. A clinical psychologist recently reported that it is 8-year-olds who show the most distress once they have absorbed the realization of death being permanent and irreversible.

From 9 years, some studies reveal a considerable interest shown in ghosts. Death is sometimes spoken of as a 'bogeyman'; children often 'play' death at school. Then by around age 12 a child's concept of death is similar to that of an adult. He will now have the added ability to see a death in terms of his own age. One boy sobbed, 'I've got to live without my daddy for about 60 years! Only Dad himself could help me do that.'

Up to adolescence, all children are far more afraid of the separation from loved people than of death itself, even their own death. And what happens afterwards is often 'heaven' or somewhere 'good and happy, with no pain', regardless of any religious background.

How to help a bereaved family

Today, many organizations have evolved to support the bereaved. Yet how many of us, whatever our status in the community, recognize our need to be more aware of how bereaved people feel? We register for first aid training; regularly give our blood – even donate parts of our bodies; join voluntary groups to help the homeless, the aged and the starving. But do we attend seminars or courses in *bereavement* counselling?

It is said that only those who have been bereaved themselves can fully understand and help others. In my experience, they are the most honest in their words of comfort. A married woman cannot know how a widow feels until her own husband dies. On the other hand, sometimes you are *unable* to understand another's sorrow because you only know your own. Your widowed friend may not feel pain in quite the way you do; her children may not miss the same things your children do. To try and help them you have first to identify *their* individual needs.

Preparation for bereavement

Parents and teachers are expected to teach children the facts of life, yet few even consider teaching them the facts of death. Due to inexperience, ignorance or fear, such an idea is dismissed as morbid, depressing or unnecessary. Certainly no prepared lesson can hope to cover all aspects of bereavement, or suit each child's circumstances. Both parents and teachers must be aware that each child has individual emotions and needs.

However, in homes and schools where the subject of death is *not* taboo, where questions are answered truthfully, where a short illness or separation is clearly explained, the whole family is far better prepared for a serious loss. Nothing can prevent shock and grief, but if a child knows that the adults in her life are easy to talk to, and receptive to confidences and problems, this fact alone can be of the greatest comfort when a tragedy occurs.

We may still shudder when reading of young children in Victorian times: when death in the family meant 'Go and help lay out Grandma in the upstairs room'; when it was not unusual for a child to see her mother dying in childbirth, or one or more brothers or sisters buried; when little children attended family funerals as regularly as weddings. Children's books, with their frequent references to dying and death, brimming with cloying sentiment or threatening hellfire and damnation, were as terrifying as any of today's horror movies.

But in the last few decades of the twentieth century was this attitude to death replaced with anything less frightening for small children? So keen were adults to protect them from such stark reality that they lapsed into a mystifying, dry-eyed silence. It became unacceptable for westerners to be 'seen' to mourn. Death, having become less familiar in childhood, became less mentionable. Like sex in Victorian times, death was now a taboo subject. Even the word was avoided: 'Jack has passed away', or 'passed on', or (more horrifying for children) 'been taken'. When a widow began to talk to her children of their father, family members and friends would change the subject. Sadly, such clumsy attempts to protect children from reality merely allowed their fantasies to grow.

As the years rolled towards the twenty-first century and there were fewer and fewer taboo subjects, feelings were expressed without embarrassment, until now even death is openly discussed, and grief recognized. Of course, we don't want a return to the days of lengthy periods of mourning, drawn curtains and sombre clothes – when even children wore black armbands on their coats – but what's so wrong with tears when someone you love has died? Your children see you laughing; let them see you crying.

Since the arrival of television, however, children are now confronted with terrifying scenes of disasters and deaths in their own living rooms – or even bedrooms. Horror movies are followed by live news flashes of war zones, suicide bombers, torture and killing. No wonder some of them cannot differentiate between reality and fiction. This means that even the words 'death', or 'dying', may conjure up sensational mind-pictures of sheer horror, of blood and slaughter. You will understand, when you read later chapters, the importance of allowing children to visit a dying relative in the quiet and peace of a hospital or hospice, and when appropriate taking them to view the tranquil sight of a laid-out body surrounded by flowers and gentle music.

Family grief

Life has to go on, but to grieve is *not* morbid, to mourn is *not* self-indulgent. A child will cope better as he grows up without a huge load of bottled-up grief weighing him down. When a tragedy happens and leaves a whole family deeply distressed and deprived, it is very natural for them all to show their grief, and very healthy if they are able to express it together. In fact, medically and emotionally, it is the safest path to take towards recovery following a bereavement.

The professionals talk of this as a 'grieving period', which can cause anxiety and prompt questions: When does it begin? Does it mean no smiles and laughter? How long will it last?

There is a danger, as a hospice social worker pointed out, of a 'language of bereavement' creeping into our literature and conversation (an unfortunate result of the growing awareness of possible serious consequences of bereavement), so that expectations of 'stages of mourning' or 'phases of grief' are held up to the newly bereaved as inevitable patterns for their future. However, a 'grieving period' simply means that no one must ever be expected to push their sadness aside and pretend that life is the same as before. We all need time in which to adapt to life without the beloved person. Perhaps it should be described more as a 'breathing space', for it will not lessen emotional shock and sadness, nor will it always stop unexpected or tragic reactions – but it can prevent the beginning of deep, inward-looking worries which could lead to psychological problems many years later.

The first task is not to protect children from their sadness – and bereavement is very, very sad. What they need is *support* during this sad time, support that includes loving and sensitive care.

How children's mourning differs from that of adults

The main difference is that a child's periods of intense grief are shorter (we've all seen tears turn to laughter in moments) but the grieving period may last much longer. 'Children get over things so quickly,' you will hear. Yet long after the adults in the family are living their changed lives with calm acceptance of a tragedy, a child can suffer despairing sadness. For as she reaches new levels of understanding, each new experience she faces arouses fresh aspects of grief: 'My first day at school made me notice all the mothers, and there I was with Daddy.'

What is 'normal' grieving?

Many families feel that too professional an approach is not right for children – they are not 'cases conforming to set patterns of bereavement behaviour'. One of my children was once treated as a 'problem child' instead of a child with a problem.

But to be aware of the emotions grief can bring, or the bizarre symptoms that might appear, *is* very comforting. For all bereaved children *do* suffer, and I for one am grateful that this is being acknowledged. They are not statistics, they are heartbroken youngsters who feel miserably let down and need to know that their bewildering emotions are natural, and that someone is trying to understand them.

It seems to me, therefore, that to know what is 'normal' is a sensible idea for anyone trying to help bereaved children. I hope the following descriptions of grief reaction will show readers that feelings such as disbelief and anger are quite usual, so that they can reassure a bereaved child with strong support and compassion, rather than say, 'Pull yourself together, dear.'

Shock

All studies agree that shock is the first response to a death, even when that death has followed a terminal illness (see Chapter 3). In adults this brings a barrage of sensations – resulting either in physical collapse or numb apathy. A child's reaction may be a silent withdrawal or a wild outburst of screaming. A very young child may feel a painful and bewildering sense of confusion rather than shock. They can't quite understand what is going on, but are sensitive to an extremely disturbed, sad atmosphere in the home, and an upset of everything familiar to them.

Distraction is not always the best policy. A baby cries, you pick her up; a toddler yells and you give him a toy or a sweet; a schoolchild is tearful and you turn on the video. Distractions work temporarily but do not alleviate the grief, merely cork it up for a bit. The medical treatment for shock is warmth and rest, and that's not a bad idea. Hug the child, let them collapse, cry, sit or lie down – don't comfort them as if they have toothache. They need time to be sad, and to talk about their mother, father, brother or sister.

Adults, while still 'in shock', are usually able to cope, albeit in a state of unreality, with the many practical affairs – notices in the paper, informing relatives and friends, arranging the funeral, etc. For children who do not have these specific things to attend to, it can become an increasingly lonely time. If they're old enough, let them take some part in the arrangements – whether that means tidying a room ready for Granny, or choosing flowers for the coffin.

Denial

William, eight, was heard telling his four-year-old brother, 'I expect Mum will come back for your birthday.' Asked if he was trying to cheer up little Jim after their mother's funeral, William grew angry and said, 'No. She may come back, how do you know she won't?'

This was no childish misunderstanding, but a very universal 'stage' of grieving – denial of the death – that is experienced by many adults in the early days of bereavement. They know their loved one is dead, may have seen his dead body, but their every thought is so centred on that person that they cannot believe he is not around. Complete 'acceptance' of a death, as it is sometimes called, may take any family a long while, and involve any of the following grief reactions.

Searching

For children this is perhaps the most logical part of their grieving. They have lost something, now they have to find it. The fact that they never do find it builds up inside them as a huge fear. 'My tummy feels excited like before Christmas, but it's a sort of terribly unhappy excitement,' was one child's very vivid description of this desolate fear of loss – a yearning that can never be fulfilled.

Ben searched so often for his daddy that he began to think of it as a game of hide and seek. His imagination grew, until one day he rushed in to his mother saying, 'Dad's come back as a ghost!' He began to visualize finding his father so distinctly that he would 'see' him in the garden or coming through a door in the house.

A child, after such an enormous loss, will be terrified of losing other people, other things – her mummy, her grandparents, her teacher, her pets and her toys. A very 'unhappy excitement' is churning round inside her.

Despair

What a tragic word. Once it is realized that no amount of searching or longing is going to find that lost person, then despair may follow. For a child, the crying may start again, the screaming and rejection of love from any other person. 'No, Mummy, I don't want you, I want Daddy!'

This is when school refusal may occur, and only love and patience can overcome this (see Chapter 7).

Anger

Even a tiny child can feel anger towards a parent who has 'left' him, or anger at a God who has 'taken' Mummy or Daddy away. 'Why didn't you make Daddy better?' 'How could you let Mummy die?' Real fury may show itself in physical toughness – perhaps breaking toys or lying kicking on the floor.

In adolescence the same anger is expressed in more out-spoken, and at times violent ways. Phil started stealing when his dad was killed on a building site. 'He used to be such a good boy,' his mother said after he was put on probation for a year. 'He's always been the loving one of the family, now he never kisses me goodnight and hits his little brothers for nothing.'

Anxiety and guilt

These 'phases' of grieving become entwined, especially for children, and seem to come under the general heading of *depression*.

A little girl is anxious about her grieving father and feels guilt that she never took her mother tea in bed that last morning. The two emotions add up to a large dose of depression.

Neil, aged 12, seemed to have survived the shock of his dad's early death, finished his searching, and worked out his anger, but was suddenly hit by overwhelming anxiety: 'I started having nightmares, my mouth was dry, I felt something awful was going to happen, every night. I kept thinking of all the things I might have done for Dad. I hated it when he asked me to cut the hedge or paint the kitchen. If I had helped him, would he have got cancer?'

Neil slumped into deep depression, and an educational psychologist was called in. This 'stage' of grief was too great to bear.

Remember also that bereaved children's minds may well be full of many practical anxieties: 'Will we still be able to go on holiday?' 'Who'll take me to school, give me my pocket money, help me with my homework?' An older child may be worried that Dad's death will mean no college, or Mum's death will mean staying at home to look after the baby.

2

Do you want to help a bereaved child?

Even with a knowledge of possible 'grief reactions', none of us can predict how we, or our children, will face a crisis until it happens. I saw my own three children, raised together, react in totally different ways when their father died suddenly one morning while they were at school.

Remember those childcare books that predict your infant's expected rate of development? 'Your baby should be dry at 18 months,' you read, and worry yourself sick as your youngest still uses 24 nappies a day. In the same way, if the bereavement therapists say your 4-year-old will suffer nightmares for six months and your 10-year-old will regress at school for a year, don't await that period with dread, it may never happen. A 10-year-old can act with heartrending adult understanding, while a 17-year-old can revert to childhood and seek dependence on a grown-up.

Sharing experiences

In Britain, Cruse Bereavement Care (see Useful addresses, page 113) has led the way in providing counselling and social support for the bereaved, and within its many branches has set up small parent circles. These create a safe and friendly setting where widowed fathers and mothers can discuss their problems, bring their children, and together learn to communicate and cope as families. Other circles have grown up among the bereaved of all ages – each trying, with the help of an empathetic and experienced 'leader', not necessarily a professional, to create a pervading atmosphere of sharing as well as caring.

Whether it is a religious, educational, cultural or social group, a small community – as further chapters will reveal – always seems to provide the most effective support for bereaved families.

I have spoken with many bereaved families in their own homes, and also in parent circles, and all agreed this to be the case. We compared the stages their children and mine have travelled through. Did they feel that knowing about the hazards en route was helpful? There were differences of opinion here, but most said that anticipating prolonged agonies of emotion, particularly in one's children, might well add extra fear to an already terrifying experience.

Many parents agonized over the behaviour of their teenagers and found it hard to assess whether this was 'normal' for adolescents or the result of the family death. One mother thought her son was turning into a delinquent after his father died.

> He started stealing from the supermarket and I was in despair until I met with another mum who said her son had stolen a car. She said the school nurse discovered the boy was upset because he couldn't drive the family car now his dad had gone. We talked it over and I realized my son worried over no pay packet coming in each week. His behaviour suddenly began to make sense.

These mothers helped each other and their frustrated sons to understand what was happening to them: 'I could never have coped alone.'

Less dramatic stories were revealed, each one giving comforting explanations of a child's anxieties. Sharing experiences seems to be the most helpful factor. 'Lindsay and me are friends 'cos we both got dads and not mums,' explained an 8-year-old at one circle I visited.

Families differ greatly about many issues – especially the benefits or otherwise of children attending funerals – but again everyone appreciated being able to discuss such subjects together.

Almost all counsellors suggest that attending the funeral is beneficial to the whole family. Apart from those with pre-school children, most parents agreed – but I heard some strong views both for and against (see Chapter 8). It was the stark, realistic descriptions of the emotions felt during grieving that brought everyone together. 'Yes, that's just how I felt,' is a familiar, relieved exclamation.

One teenager described how coming out of her initial, numbed shock felt 'like coming round from an anaesthetic'. Another girl thought it was like being knocked out. The two girls probably hadn't told anyone of their feelings, but now they could share, now they were not alone.

Not all children's grief is visible – some suffer *all* the possible phases, some only one or two of them. None of the children I met 'went through' them at the same time, or in the same way. Shock in one meant silence, in another weeping; anger in one meant turning your sister's bedroom upside down, in another it meant excessive rudeness to your teacher. Numbness, yearning and searching did not always appear, and many said guilt was never a problem. There was certainly no 'time limit' to each phase.

Those who have never experienced bereavement talk of grief 'coming to an end'. 'Are you over it all now?' they ask of your children, as though they had been suffering from measles. Grief is never 'over'; we learn to travel through it, and it is up to us to help our children to travel with us. If we keep memories alive for them it will help to create a positive aspect to their grieving, and eventually strengthen them in their journey through life.

A great deal does depend on the family situation before the tragedy, and on the relationships within that family. We all cope with death very much as we do with life. It also depends on the support available immediately after the tragedy occurs.

Death of a grandparent

Often this is the first major bereavement in a child's life. Even when a grandparent has never been a great part of the family's life, a child will learn something of the consequences of death from her parent's grief reactions. When the children have lived with a grandparent – if their mother goes to work, or has been divorced, or is tied to a handicapped sibling – the impact of such a death is particularly strong. The two-generation gap can, strangely, make this an extremely close relationship. Parents sometimes ignore a child's sorrow, being too sad themselves at *their* parent's death; it has been known for parents not to tell children the news until after the grandparent's funeral has taken place; and teachers may ridicule a request for a child to be excused from school after her grandmother has died.

The grieving may not be as long-lasting as that following a parent's or sibling's death, but it should never be ignored. An understanding idea would be to let a child choose something tangible as a memento – her grandfather's watch, or her grandmother's special photo album. One little girl took over the feeding of her granny's cat, and a teenage boy looked after his granddad's vegetable garden: 'I know he'd not want it to be wasted.'

But the questions will still be asked: 'If Granny (or Granddad) *is* in heaven, how come she (he) is buried?' After a grandfather has died, often the image of his old jacket can be used. 'Granddad's body was rather like an old coat, wasn't it? Not much use to him any more, so he's left it behind for us to bury.'

Breaking the news

Children's perception of death is often confused (see page 1), and having to tell a child of a loved person's death is probably the hardest thing any adult has to face. Obviously, the person closest to the child, either the surviving parent, an older brother or sister, will be the best person. But a parent may be too shocked to be coherent, or the child may be some distance away. Then whoever is the most familiar and trusted adult to that child will have to tell her the news.

Whatever age the child is, take her in your arms, hold her hand, or hug her on your lap – touch is all-important, and the most comforting sensation in times of crisis. In a hospital waiting room a father was seen to walk in and tell his 7-year-old daughter that her mother had died. He never even took her hand. It was a nurse who had to reach out to that child. Your loving presence, your compassion and ability to tell the child you love her, that her dead parent loved her and that she will never be abandoned – these are the feelings and atmosphere she will carry inside her for the rest of her life.

Tears may or may not follow: shock is a shattering emotion and can stifle crying for a while. Whether there is silence, screaming and weeping, or unbelieving questioning, listen to the child, and provide as much reassurance as you can, honestly. 'Yes, Mummy was badly hurt.' 'No, it was not your fault that Jimmy had an accident when he was riding your bike.' Children readily assume blame for a family death and need repeated assurances that they are not guilty in any way.

Emily, aged 6, was given no such comfort. One day after school she found her mother and teenage sister crying in the kitchen. Without a word, they took Emily upstairs to see her father lying dead in bed. The shocked little girl had an overwhelming sense of guilt. 'I thought I had done it!' The day before, her father had been gardening and had come indoors saying he was tired and wanted a glass of water. Emily was sent to fetch one. And now in her bewildered little mind, she thought that the glass of water had caused his death. 'No one explained anything. I don't even remember anyone giving me a hug or a kiss.'

Children frequently fear death for themselves also. 'Is cancer catching?' 'Will I die when I'm 15 as well?' Such fears are very real, and should never be dismissed with scorn, anger, or a laugh.

Many children will be overwhelmed by anger. You brought them this devastating news, so they may vent that anger on you. 'I hate you, you're a liar, I want my mother!'

The anger and denial will tumble out along with the shock, and this is not the time to argue. A family therapist advised, 'Don't ask a child to postpone, deny, or cover up her feelings. Grief that is postponed can return months or even years later to haunt the child.'

Some older children prefer to be alone. The adult side of their personality will make them long to get right away, perhaps run through fields or along a beach, maybe shut themselves in a room to play a guitar, or walk around the town until they are physically exhausted. Never criticize or argue with them; their behaviour is natural and can be extremely therapeutic.

The person who will be most valued in any bereaved household is not one offering buckets of sympathy, but one who is unobtrusively 'around', quietly getting on with everyday tasks, taking phone calls, answering doorbells, giving children their supper, feeding the cat, or lighting the boiler. Listen to the children if they seem forgotten and want to talk. Be careful, however, not to 'take over' a household and leave the family to sit staring at each other. Being occupied is an acknowledged therapy in many traumatic situations.

Less helpful is the person who tries to burden a child with immediate adult responsibilities. Jack was only 8 when told by his uncle, 'You're the man now, don't upset your mother by crying.' Holding back his tears was not only unnatural, but dangerous for that little boy. Luckily, he saw several men, including his grandfather, openly crying at his father's funeral, and was able to mourn with his mother.

On the other hand, Tanya told me that her father died when she was 14, and she found herself unable to weep after the first day. 'All the family cried so much, I felt ashamed. I remember rubbing my eyes to make them red so everyone would think I'd been crying on the day of the funeral.'

A counsellor commented, 'Yes, this can happen. Probing can be unhelpful, and therapists who "try to make you cry" are too clinical to be of any real help. They can be resented, even laughed at by intelligent adults and teenagers.'

In trying to help a family where a parent is too overwhelmed by grief to notice if a child needs special attention, take care not to separate the family; it's important that they share their feelings as much as possible. Never, except perhaps for a tiny baby, be tempted to 'whisk the children away'. Decisions taken must always include the whole family, but a child therapist stressed that you have to guard against advocating treatments and handing out advice towards young children simply because 'that's the thing to do', or 'that's what my mother did'. The best advice to helpers I ever heard came from a young nurse: 'Help with your heart.'

How to get children to talk

Counsellors always advise getting children to talk of their worries. This is not always easy. You may have a good rapport with a child, yet he seldom asks you a direct question. You wish you could help him to say what is at the back of his mind. A consultant child psychiatrist said:

> Even we psychiatrists can't read people's minds. But because a child has been referred due to bereavement, we can safely assume the sentence in his mind will involve something he wishes he had said to his parent. Ask the child if this is so. He will welcome your understanding.

Another sensitive child therapist said:

> Their needs seem very obvious, but only recently have adults come to see that they need recognition of their pain and fear in

an insecure world, and a chance to express their feelings about death and about the person they have lost.

She added that strong grief need not destroy a family, but can often bond it.

On a practical level, try to keep a family's routine as unchanged as possible. If Dad had provided pocket money, see that it's continued; if Mum always made sandwiches for school, get the children to help you make them; if dancing class or football practice is on Saturday morning, try to ensure the youngsters are taken there on time.

Bereavement is often considered 'over' after the funeral. Dad or Mum goes back to work, children to school, the family is expected to be 'back to normal'. Now is the time when an absence will be most deeply felt – life seems strangely far from normal.

In the early days of bereavement, it helps children to know that there are no right or wrong feelings. How you, their parent or carer, feel is what matters and you must never be afraid to express what you feel. As the weeks go by, children may develop minor ailments – sore throats, aching limbs – especially if their parent died of an illness. Many start biting their nails, wetting the bed, stammering, or become lethargic, overtired and unable to sleep. None of these symptoms is a cause for immediate alarm, but should be watched (see pages 20–1 for more advice).

There are no specific ways of helping each individual problem, but if you appreciate that each one is caused by a deep sorrow and a need for love and attention, then you will probably find practical solutions as you go along. For example, if a child refuses her food, perhaps helping you to cook will stimulate an interest. 'What about making some gingerbread men for Linda?' can encourage an older child to help cheer up a younger sister.

Constant aggressive behaviour and bad temper is infuri-ating, and a grieving, overtired parent can be pushed to her limits. 'When the doctor said I shouldn't punish them, I could have screamed. How much can I let them get away with?' An anguished mother voiced her very natural feelings at a parents' circle where several mothers and fathers were full of sympathy. So what's the answer? Even family members cannot always tell how much bad behaviour is due to the present crisis. Children have admitted later to crying, hitting and spitting 'just to get sympathy'.

One young widow found that providing her small children with play blocks, cardboard boxes, tough brown paper, balloons, and other objects suitable for banging, tearing and breaking, enabled them to rid themselves of a lot of venom. But what about the older children? 'I felt like sending mine down to the carbreaker's yard,' said one frantic father, and he had the right idea. If you live in the country, activities like digging ditches, clearing hedges, cutting branches, and plenty of cycle rides can help; and in town, painting, carpentry or cleaning cars for pocket money is better than standing on street corners or going to the cinema.

A family therapist with wide experience suggests discussing with a child the ultimate outcome of his aggressive behaviour – in other words, acknowledging it rather than complaining about it. Show them, she says, that:

> It is normal to be filled with anger at such an irreversible loss. But that no amount of screaming, wailing, punching or kicking is going to bring back that loved person – and so using up the violent feelings in other physical ways is a sensible thing to do.

This sounds fine in theory; it needs to be put across to a distraught child with empathy and conviction – and the idea may be rejected. But it's worth a try, and in families of several children it may lead to healthy competition: 'I can get rid of more anger than you!' And if a parent can explain that he or she is full of anger too, it often helps. After all, this whole tragedy is a family crisis, shared by every member.

I would suggest that during the early months after bereavement, you look on a child who appears to be having more difficulty handling the situation than his brothers and sisters as one with a handicap. Let him know that you appreciate his problem, and want to help, but at the same time don't be tempted to spoil him and treat him differently from the other children – let him see he can't get away with everything. Deep inside himself, he doesn't want to be different, but wants to know that someone understands.

Apart from the grief, whether it is a parent or a sibling who has died, the household is going to be altered. The secure home a child has known is threatened; he finds it difficult to trust anyone now, and the future looks bleak. For a start, he has to get used to strangers saying, 'Where's your dad?' or 'Is your mum at home?' It is not at all unusual for the reply to be, 'She's out.'

For many months, probably up to the first anniversary of the death, there will be periods when strong emotions will abound and often overshadow all the normally happy occasions such as birthdays and Christmas. After that time, these emotional outbursts usually lessen. The loss is not forgotten, but the family will have learned to handle it.

When does a child need professional help?

Many parents shudder at the idea of an educational psychologist, or any kind of psychiatric treatment. There is a curious stigma attached even to child guidance clinics. Any referral suggests inability to handle your own children; it hints of abnormality in the family; what will the neighbours say? 'No shrinks for us, thank you.'

Conversely, some parents rush to refer their child at the first sign of unusual behaviour, when it is *they* who need treatment. However, as with physical illness, early signs of inability to cope with bereavement are far better diagnosed and treated immediately than left to smoulder until they burst into flame in adult life (see Chapter 10).

The signs to watch out for are continued uncontrolled behaviour, intense vulnerability even to small separations, or – a sign often ignored – a complete absence of *any* show of feelings. If a parent says, 'Sally is quite over it, never gives us any trouble,' that's when a careful watch is needed over the little girl.

In teenagers, watch for anorexia, severe insomnia and hallucinations. A psychiatrist says, 'Adolescents take life more seriously than they are given credit for, and their depression is often anger turned inwards. If this is not recognized, it may turn to blind rage, as they feel increasingly abandoned.'

I asked him how a parent can know if a child's grief is becoming 'pathological', when emotions become distorted. He summed up his advice: 'Watch for grief that is delayed, prolonged or strangely disturbed.' And he also confirmed that 'You must take equally seriously grief that is absent.'

Where to go for help

The wisest course to take for a child who seems 'stuck' in his grieving is to speak with your family doctor. He or she may be able to give experienced guidance initially, but more often you will be referred to a child guidance clinic, which will decide if a child is seriously in need of psychiatric help.

If you have joined a widows' or other bereavement counselling organization, you may find other families willing to introduce you to specialists they have found helpful. This is an ideal way to find the right therapist for your child – as with a doctor or dentist, there can be personality clashes, and it is essential that a child is comfortable with the professional chosen.

At any age, a child may be reluctant to attend his first appointment, and great care must be taken to assure him that he is not ill, or 'different'. Many children, however, are quietly pleased that someone has noticed their difficulty in coping with these weird emotions they are experiencing. They may not admit this, or even appear grateful, but I can assure you they will appreciate your concern.

The psychiatrist will probably wish to see the parent/s on the first visit, but after that it is usual for the child to be seen alone. As with adults, talking with a stranger can release many inhibitions, and as long as a rapport is achieved, then many tensions that have been strangling your child's feelings will be loosened and he will find his self-esteem restored. Afterwards, he may not be able to tell you what was said, or why he feels any different. Don't pressure him to tell you – he will be welcoming this one-to-one discussion. If the relationship has been good, he may well be reluctant to stop the sessions – can he manage alone? A good clinical psychiatrist will know when the child can cope, and will also assure him that he can return any time he wants to discuss further problems. One psychiatrist told me that children often contact him up to two years afterwards if they have to face any crisis.

Similarly, if you are a parent, carer, teacher or priest helping a child to mourn, you will find a time comes when you can both move on to other things. But the bond between you will be strong, and you must make sure that child can always find you in future when she needs extra reassurance and support.

Children needing extra help

If there is a mentally handicapped child in the family, never underestimate their ability to understand what has occurred or the depth of their emotions. They need to be as closely involved in the mourning as other children, and given extra signs of love and support.

3

Terminal illness

Many children are actively excluded from the knowledge of a parent's or sibling's fatal illness, in the mistaken belief that this will protect them from pain and suffering. The result is that, amid obvious distress and disruption, terrifying fantasies can build up:

> My mother took two years to die. I was never told of the seriousness of her illness, but I must have sensed it. I used to get panics, and thought if I became a mother I'd also have to stay in bed all the time. When she actually died I don't remember being told, everyone just assumed that I knew. It was the day before my tenth birthday, and I thought I'd be put in an orphanage.

Certainly the drawn out agony of terminal illness is no easier to bear than the trauma of sudden, perhaps violent, death. But once that illness is acknowledged, and the nursing of it shared by the patient's family, the preparation for dying and bereavement can be a gradual process.

When children should be told

Ideally, when a fatality strikes, the children should be included in a family discussion, told what is happening (in relation to their ages and understanding) and not left alone with their fears and sorrow. They can then share in both the responsibilities that arise and the mourning. Many families manage wonderfully, help each other, talk and cry together, continue to live as normally as possible in the circumstances. But for others it is a time of lonely anxiety. All families know that you recover from measles or tonsillitis – but an illness from which you never recover is unthinkable, and therefore unmentionable. 'I was 11 when my mother told me I must spend Easter with my cousins. I never asked her why and when I came home three weeks later Mum told me Dad was dead.'

This boy's sadness at losing his adored daddy would not have been lessened if his mother had had the courage to tell him the truth. But he might have had that precious chance to say goodbye, and not felt the added trauma of being 'left out' of the family circle.

Terminal illness in a home creates its own, devastating difficulties, both emotional and practical, not least of which is trying to supply the children with consistent, realistic information. I am not suggesting that telling children that a parent or sibling is dying is going to eliminate all problems. But it *can* start a sort of anticipatory grieving process, a preparation time, which has been known to ease slightly the bereavement to come. In other words, the idea of death is introduced gradually: 'Mummy has an illness from which some people die.' Older children will learn the meaning of the word terminal. Some fears, anger and anguish may be eliminated, and what Freud termed 'grief work' may start even before the parent dies.

A 12-year-old girl found the right words to describe this traumatic time in her life:

> I felt sorry for myself when I heard Mum had leukaemia, which I knew was a life-threatening illness; but then I saw how sick she was and felt sorry for *her*. Long illness doesn't hurt less than sudden death, it just helps you to withstand the pain of the loss better.

Hearing the diagnosis

Hearing that an illness is fatal usually brings similar responses to news of a death – shock, numbness, disbelief and denial. Then come fear, anxiety, helplessness and anger: Why me? Why her? Why us? It can bring resentment towards others who are well, and sometimes guilt at one's own health. Told that his days are numbered, a parent may well be bitter, irritable, difficult to live with. Told that her child is dying, a mother may withdraw with numb despair: Why her, not me?

In this suddenly changed atmosphere, children may feel jealous of the attention and sympathy received by the patient. A small child may behave badly and so become more alienated. On being told, 'Be quiet, you'll make Daddy worse,' his belief in his ability to make wishes come true can be strengthened. Why shouldn't the fatal prognosis on a father or sister be magically changed by his behaviour?

A girl of 15 thought her own difficult birth had caused her mother's cancer. She was never given help to understand the reality of terminal illness, and having no one to talk with after her mother's death, built up a wall of isolating guilt for many years.

However honest you are with younger children, your words can easily be misinterpreted: 'Daddy had a heart attack' conjures up a physical attack – which to a child with a vivid imagination could have been performed with an axe, or even by a gang of terrorists. Less horrific, but equally confusing, was a little girl's reaction on being told her granny had died from a stroke: 'But I stroked the cat and she didn't die.'

Hospital care

Parents sometimes argue that 'hospital is not a place for children', and for some I would agree. If your parent is lying in a huge ward surrounded by oxygen cylinders and drip feeds, among bleeping monitors, endless groans or harsh breathing, it can be terrifying. The firm criteria must surely be that pre-school children are not dragged in on every visit, but left with familiar and trusted carers, and kept well informed according to their level of understanding.

Children in hospital

Despite their often grim exteriors, hospitals for children are a world away from the Dickensian atmosphere of isolation our grandparents suffered. Bright colours, noisy wards, toys, visiting children running around, and an overwhelming sense of caring, provide all possible comfort to the whole family. At last, hospital staff understand that a mother's hug can be as beneficial as a week's supply of junior aspirin.

Traditionally, hospitals and doctors have no answers for the dying – medicine is about curing, and if it fails they are at a loss to know what to do. However, changing attitudes in recent years place far more emphasis on the wider needs of patients and their families. A much broader curriculum for nursing training has been started by the English National Board for nursing, which includes 'counselling' and 'adjustment to loss', and definite, compulsory training in bereavement care; the Board considers this aspect of the training very important. Young nurses can gain practical experience in counselling skills along with their medical expertise, either within a hospice or with a home care team. In particular, those entering sick children's nursing, paediatrics or school nursing are encouraged to discuss their own feelings and reactions to dying and death.

Nurses are seldom likely to be left alone with a bereaved family, and many hospitals have psychiatrists available to support them on the wards.

Training for medical students is also broadening in its outlook. A child psychologist on the staff of a large teaching hospital says that work on the wards does not only include patient care. Doctors nowadays appreciate that 'visiting relatives may need us as much as the patients do', and they are now taught to deal sympathetically with anxious questions.

Teaching hospitals often host speakers from all counselling sources to conduct seminars on areas such as 'children's concepts of death', 'helping children grieve', and other relevant themes. As a result, many doctors realize that they could be more sensitive in their reactions. All doctors need to appreciate that dying and death are 'family affairs' and that caring for a bereaved family is essentially a preventive form of medical care.

Hospice care

St Christopher's Hospice in the south of England, started by Dame Cicely Saunders for the care of the terminally ill, is now internationally known, and the hospice movement is spreading throughout the world. Basically, it appreciates that dying patients need dignity, peace and understanding as well as medical and nursing skills.

Doctors and staff do not wear white coats; a nurse told me they have never had a small child refuse to come in, however great their grief. As one little girl said, 'Sadness *hurts*, Mummy.' But at least hospice care takes the mystique out of illness and death, and that can only be good. The pervading atmosphere is of caring; no one is allowed to feel a burden to anyone else. In a hospice a nurse sitting chatting on a patient's bed is *working*.

The whole family is involved. A small boy whose father was dying was found playing chess with a grandmother whose daughter was dying. They shared feelings and consolation.

In England, there are now several hospices run specifically for children – but ill and dying children need to be near home. The further they are away from their parents the less likely they are to relax. They are far more afraid of *separation* from their parents than of dying itself. So most hospitals have a local children's unit, run very much on the family-oriented lines of a hospice.

In one specialist hospice unit for dying children, the nurses and social workers take special interest in the visiting brothers and sisters – and know them all by name. They are invaluable in helping parents prepare themselves and their children for bereavement. As one hospice social worker said: 'Parents often whisper to me that there are certain things the children must not hear, must not be told. But when all the family gather for a discussion, who asks all the leading questions? The youngest child, invariably.'

One or more highly qualified social workers, with experience in family and group therapy, psychiatric work and/or bereavement therapy, is normally attached to a hospice. They can liaise with outside social workers, doctors and district nurses, and with the hospice professionals. Their role in helping families is unique on a practical and emotional level, both before and after bereavement.

Of course, it is not all sweetness and light, all calm and acceptance. Many of those involved refuse to accept the terminal diagnosis. Many families have spent months of struggling at home with pain and fear, endless treatments, sleepless nights; entering a hospice is seen as a sort of 'giving up'. Children quickly sense this despair and bitterness and wonder what is happening. A teenager who came home from school one day to find his mother had been moved to a hospice was horrified. 'That's where people go to die! You can't send Mum there!'

But once a hospice team takes over, tension eases, people relax. More importantly, the families know they can talk and someone will listen.

The moment of death

When children themselves are dying, they often seem more concerned about their parents than what is going to happen to them. Nurses are constantly asked, 'Please look after Mummy and Daddy,' but not, 'Where am I going?' or 'Will it be all right?' Their healthy brothers and sisters seem more concerned about whether death will be painful.

Where possible, the whole family will be present when the patient dies. Hospice staff try to be discreet and sensitive – bodies are never whisked away too quickly, and families are encouraged to visit the dead person afterwards.

How different from the doctor who said to two schoolchildren, 'You don't want to see your daddy now he's dead, do you?' What an appalling, negative question for grief-stricken children. Of course, it is entirely up to the family and the children – none of us knows how we will react. One teenager was 'shocked at seeing Granny, she looked so old and ugly'. Another said, 'I'll always remember Mum lying there – I can't get her unsmiling face out of my mind.'

I feel strongly that future memories are all-important for children, and that those of mother, father, sister or brother should be of those precious people *very much alive*. Yet one boy of 14 found that 'It helped me to accept that my brother really had died,' and many families are grateful afterwards that they had this time to say goodbye.

Television scenes of violent deaths can haunt both children and adults – but seeing a small room with floral curtains and vases of flowers, where the beloved family member is lying covered in a softly coloured blanket, is a lasting picture far removed from the appalling images of screen deaths in sterile mortuaries.

Death still comes as a shock. The reality is always more traumatic than the anticipation. However 'well prepared' they are, children will be shattered by their feelings: 'I was sick in the garden.' 'I couldn't stop shaking.'

The remarks of neighbours and acquaintances can be unintentionally insensitive. 'Well, it was expected, dear.' Expected it may have been but it is still a huge tragedy, as agonizing as if she had been in a car crash. Your mum is dead.

Ambivalent feelings may follow later. After a long illness, with many hospital admissions and the difficulties they have brought, a feeling of relief creeps in, which may add guilt to a child's sorrow.

Many families find their greatest comfort in each other. 'I remember the nights we all used to wander down to the kitchen if we couldn't sleep,' says Anne, whose husband died when her son was 14 and her daughter 16. 'We chatted, often cried, and at times found ourselves cutting honey sandwiches and laughing – we were together, and that seemed to help.'

This natural ability to handle a crisis is within so many people, and it would be a backward step if bereavement counselling – excellent and necessary as it is in many instances – were to intrude on that self-healing within strong family groups.

Sadly, not all families are strong, or united, and many have difficulties even before bereavement hits them, which inevitably confuse their reactions (see Chapter 9).

Going home to die

With terminal illness, the professionals are now realizing that science must not blind them to compassion and that what they *could* do is not necessarily what they *should* do. Once curative treatment has stopped and symptom control been established, the hospital or hospice always hopes that families will feel supported enough to allow patients, especially children, to die at home, and not feel abandoned. Being included in the preparation for the family death and in the process of bereavement has considerable benefits. Of course, parents will now need strong support, not least in answering questions like, 'Why didn't the hospital make Sally better?'

In an increasing number of areas, home care teams are available day and night to help. In Britain, Macmillan nurses specialize in caring for cancer patients in their own homes. There may be dissension in the family over the decision: grandparents in particular may feel that a parent dying at home is too much for a young family to bear; others may feel that the experience helps children to grow and mature.

Even in homes that are not 'ideal' – where the family members quarrel or fight, and are less than sensitive towards children – it is still the place where everyone can be themselves, where young people feel safe surrounded by familiar things.

The bereaved are not forgotten

Children's hospital and hospice wards do not always end their care with the death of the patient. They recognize that death and bereavement are not two separate things. Home care teams can supply great support by visiting a family for some weeks after the funeral. It is nearly a year since little Toby died, yet his former nurse still visits his family and takes little sister Jane on outings. She knows how vital the continuation of a friendship is to a young child.

Teenagers and bereavement

Children in their late teens will sometimes refuse to visit a parent or sibling in the hospice. For the adolescent, cosy explanations just don't work any more. The fact that his mother is in a hospice means that she is going to die. He is angry at the doctors for not making her better; he is angry that *he* is not the centre of this family drama; he may even be angry at feeling this way. Sadly, bitterness and guilt build up when he finds out how he has disappointed his family.

For at this difficult time in his life, an adolescent will be trying to find and assert himself as a person *apart* from his parents – he will rebel against doing anything, from shopping to visiting friends 'with Mum and Dad'. At the same time he is afraid that at a hospital bedside he will be expected to behave like a grown-up, and he knows he is still no good at 'saying the right thing' – ambivalent feelings indeed.

Hospice staff, with their wide experience of young people, have many suggestions. Never 'take' your child along on a duty visit. Suggest that he calls in on his way home from school and you'll meet him in the hall (sometimes it is that first walk into the building that he finds so hard). 'Pop in for five minutes,' would be a sensible idea, or ask your teenager to bring something in that their ill parent needs. 'Leave it at the desk if you like.' Make things as low-key as possible.

Most teenagers will be surprised to find that the staff appear *un*threatening, and probably far easier to talk with than their own families, which helps them to face this new and frightening experience. A social worker stressed how valuable a teenager can be within a family: 'They are so knowledgeable today, often understanding the scientific workings of a modern hospital far better than their parents.'

One excellent idea, started by St Christopher's Hospice and now being taken up by many others, brings together teenagers who have lost a parent into a group where youngsters can meet and talk freely. There is no counselling unless requested. Teenagers need to be part of a peer group. They do not want to be 'talked at' by adults, at a time when they are trying to break free of parental bonds. So if one parent dies their emotions are extremely complex. 'How can I break away now when I'll have to look after Mum?' 'Do you think Dad will marry again?'

At first, they are suspicious of such a group, but once they start talking, unhampered by parents or teachers hovering over them, they discover many feelings in common, and often sort out problems for each other. Conversations pour out, some painful, some negative, but all helping the teenagers to find out that their frightening, tangled thoughts are not unusual.

4

Unexpected death

'In the morning I had a dad. At suppertime he was gone, and our family was one person short.' The 15-year-old girl summed up the stark, stupendous impact of a sudden death. No human being can absorb news that a loved person, who was talking, eating, sleeping or laughing with them only hours previously is now *not alive*.

Shock promotes urgent and fierce denial in adults, causes disbelief in an older child, and despair in a tiny child. At any age the news of an unexpected death – due to sudden illness, accident, or violence – brings similar feelings of helplessness to the survivors.

It is understandable, then, that an adult's instinct is to protect a child from this agony. Sometimes information is withheld, or delayed. 'Mummy's not well, dear, you must stay with me.' Kindly meant, but instead of supplying preparation time for that child to adjust to bereavement, false news brings fear and anxiety.

Parents frequently hide the truth, and not only from their youngest children. Bob's father went into hospital for a minor operation and died under the anaesthetic. His mother couldn't bring herself to tell her intelligent 9-year-old son, who worshipped his father. Three days later, when friends finally told him about his father, his grief was overwhelmed by anger at not being told the truth. He never spoke of this, but became withdrawn at home and troublesome at school. Not until five years later did he finally break down when talking to an understanding teacher. He cried and shouted, and it all came pouring out: 'I wasn't told for three days.'

That teacher spoke from years of caring experience:

Children often cope better than their parents ... I find it's essential to keep them busy, give them plenty to do. Well-meaning friends tend to think it kind to relieve them of any work – but physical and mental exercise is the best therapy. Children *can* cope with tragedy, face up to responsibilities, *if they know the truth*. But it is essential that their own strength is backed up by the support of a loving family.

Violent and sudden death

Bob lost his dad suddenly, with no warning. But the cause of the death was illness. Would a violent accident or a vicious killing cause more shock, and be even more difficult to comprehend and to bear?

Colleen was only 3 when her father was killed on a pedestrian crossing. Sue, her broken-hearted young mother, did not tell her little girl immediately:

When her great-granny had died, we said she had gone to heaven, and Colleen kept asking us to drive her there. So what could I tell her now? I left it until she asked me herself. She cried at first, but seemed more upset about a little friend whose mum was single and had *never* had a daddy ... Now, at 5, Colleen often gets out of bed during the night to check I'm still there. She fantasizes a lot, exaggerates the happiness of life with Daddy. She gets upset playing with other families when the dad's at home. 'My daddy's dead,' she tells them.

Teenagers' experience

Joan was 17 and her sister Linda 12 when their lives were shattered following a knock on their front door one evening:

Mum answered the door and we heard a policeman telling her that Daddy had had a heart attack in his car and was dead. I heard myself sort of wail, and Linda let out a scream. I cried and cried, although not really believing it. I was a bit of a painful teenager. I wasn't getting on well with Mum and Dad – nothing serious but I kept flaring up. I felt guilty, yet couldn't stop being bad-tempered and irritable. We went to the funeral. I hated it, somehow it was so final, but I'm glad I went. It's almost like you can start again after that.

Linda was worried about her mother: 'It made me think about death. I felt sick if mum was late home from work.'

'I saw Mummy die'

Even more disturbing are the accidents in which children see their parent/s die. Jim was 7 when his mother and twin brother were killed in a car crash. He escaped with a bruised hand, but suffered huge guilt along with his grief. He had always been the 'naughty' one of the family, and frequently been told to 'sit still on the back seat or Mummy will have an accident'. For months the little boy was silent, his only defence against his strong feelings of sadness. It was several years before a doctor helped his father to talk over young Jim's fears and absolve him from his load of guilt.

Thirteen-year-old Don was in a car that skidded down a hillside, killing his father and seriously injuring his mother. Miraculously, he was thrown clear. Unlike Jim, he has never suffered guilt feelings, but admits that all emotions seem to have been stifled since that day: 'The only time I cried was at the funeral when they were putting Dad in the hole, and that was because my grandparents were very upset. And now I don't react to traumas whatever the pressure.'

Don's obvious denial, as the experts would describe it, of his father's death, does seem to have enabled him to cope with his life since the accident. Now a father himself, he says, 'The actual death must not be allowed to stimulate a change of behaviour for life.'

A 12-year-old American girl was the only survivor in a car crash that killed both her parents, and her brother and sister. A tragic story – could any child survive such shock and grief?

Initially it caused her not only acute denial, but an attempt to keep her family completely outside her memory.

Surely at her age she could not be expected to cope with her devastating loss without help? She was sent to live with relatives, where her unspoken grief showed in appalling behaviour problems:

I wasn't sad. I was in a weird sort of state, not caring what happened to me. I kept thinking this is a dream, I shall soon be home and nothing will have changed. I thought like that for about three or four years.

Finally she spent six months in a psychiatric hospital, but it still took a long while before she would talk:

I used to fight them off (literally, I was violent at times) and once ended up in a straitjacket at a group therapy session. Eventually I let it all out. I sort of got my whole head straightened out, now I feel in control. I know that anything I do I'm responsible for ... I learned that you can't sit there and mourn ... If you want to help young people who are bereaved encourage them to talk. They may need pushing – and don't ever push too soon – for talking may cause them a lot of pain ... stay calm and listen, never judge, that's what children want.

Suicide

Although without doubt the most traumatic of sudden deaths – bringing shock, horror, remorse, guilt, shame and confusion to survivors – suicide is not always totally unexpected. Many depressive illnesses, for example, can be thought of as 'terminal'; as such their termination is often from suicide.

Doctors and nurses can and do help families of mentally ill patients to acknowledge the illness as 'a sickness of the mind'. My own doctor helps parents explain this to their children by saying, 'Mummy has a special sickness in her mind. Her thinking and feeling is painful, that's why you can't see it, there's no sickness on the outside of her body.'

However, while death may be the last taboo topic of conversation in western society, suicide beats it for the shame, stigma and mystery that still follow in its wake, even in our supposedly enlightened century. Because of this people don't, often won't, talk about it except perhaps in whispers. All of this may prompt a surviving parent to tell the children nothing at all, or else lie to them.

Suicide, no matter what its cause, is not easy to explain to a child, any more than is a parent's desertion through divorce, without making that child feel abandoned. 'A sort of reject, not wanted,' was how one child described her immediate feelings. Certainly, very special difficulties arise. In all families, the varied and tragic consequences of a parent's suicide are magnified by the withholding, or distortion, of the truth.

Sally was 10 when her father killed himself:

> I remember everybody crying. Lucy and me – she was 5 – sort of guessed Dad had died, but I don't think anyone told us. Whenever I asked, Mum got angry, and I found Gran putting away all Dad's photos so I didn't dare ask *her*. My teacher changed towards me, hardly took any notice of me, I felt ostracized somehow. All grown-ups seemed to whisper a lot. What was the awful secret about Daddy? Six years later, the night before I went away to college, Mummy told me Daddy had shot himself as he'd done something wrong at his office and was ashamed. She told me not to tell anyone.

It was years before Sally could even begin to understand an adult's pain and misery that could cause him to leave his loving family.

For many families, guilt becomes the overwhelming part of their anguish. Christine said her mother often shouted at her and her brother: 'You two will drive me crazy!' Later, after her mother had overdosed, Christine overheard a doctor talking about 'that crazy woman'. Is it surprising that, at 13, the young girl's burden of blame started years of severe depression?

Cynthia's two daughters were teenagers when their father

threw himself under a train, and they had completely opposite reactions:

> My 14-year-old cried all day on hearing the news, but then nothing. She calmly took on the mantle of looking after me and her sister; her only sign of grief was to visit her father's grave once a week. But my 15-year-old grew deeply depressed and took a mild overdose. She wouldn't eat, and would only wear black. She became very disturbed, her memory of the events becoming distorted, and she kept yelling things that were untrue. One day she shouted, 'If it wasn't for you, Daddy would still be here.' Finally she agreed to see a behaviour therapist, and slowly improved. We still have to tread carefully with her, her room is full of mementoes of her daddy, and her diary is locked.

Cynthia is a brave lady who recognized her daughter's anger was part of her grief and shock, and not personal bitterness towards her mother.

I welcome the professionals' awareness of children's suffering in these tragedies. Their studies, however, should only be read by the various caring professions. One family, following the schizophrenic father's dramatic suicide, were given an expert's book 'to help us through'. It contained stark, shocking statements on parental suicide, such as 'Daughters of paternal suicide will never be able to form satisfactory relationships with men', and little on the causes of suicide.

That family had the sense to get rid of the book before it added to their misery and guilt. Plenty of academic literature exists on these lines – all well researched and undoubtedly disturbing in its findings – but it is *not* suitable for bereaved families without guidance from understanding professionals.

What is shocking is that more and more children, many not yet in their teens (the youngest recorded, in the United States, being 7 years old), are committing suicide. In Britain, the suicide rate for teenagers has risen steadily in the last half-century. Sadly, some *are* due to family bereavement, and the experts list four reasons for such tragic reactions:

1 They wish to be reunited with the dead person.
2 They want revenge against him/her.
3 They wish to destroy themselves to assuage guilt feelings.
4 They feel life is not worth living without that person.

Stephen, at 15, explained his reasons:

> Dad and me had an argument, and I slammed out of the house
> and went to stay with a friend. A week later Dad died, had a heart
> attack in bed. When I got home I hated the house without him;
> if only I could tell him I loved him. Then at the funeral I realized
> I *could* tell him if I could die and meet him again like the priest
> said.

Luckily, Stephen's attempt at suicide failed, and his mother and
a counsellor friend finally made the boy believe that his father
loved him and knew his true feelings. It took a long time.

Attempted suicides

Many children make frequent suicide 'gestures' – cries for help,
for some loving care and attention. These often follow family
suicide, but are also understandable in situations where a child
is living in chaotic and unstable circumstances, ill-treated, or
simply neglected.

Conversely, one teenager told me that for her, the 'option of
suicide' was taken away by her father's death.

> Up till then, suicide seemed a wonderfully dramatic thing to
> do – you know how emotional teenagers can be! But when I real-
> ized how much grief a family death can cause, I knew I could
> never inflict further suffering on my mother and sisters.

When children need psychiatric help

Some situations are so horrific, that children cannot be expected
to cope without help. When a family member has been a murder
victim, then hate and terror are added to a child's emotions –
their lives are shattered.

Julian, aged 16, came home one day to find his father had hanged himself; a little girl of 10 saw her mother jump out of the window to her death. Not surprisingly, evidence suggests that psychiatric disturbance following such witnessing of a parent's suicide is unusually high, often taking the form of anxiety or misbehaviour. A leading child psychiatrist said:

> Children usually come to see me at least a year or two after bereavement, especially following a violent death. It usually means that something significant at the time was handled imperfectly, or wasn't done, or talked about. When bereavement is from suicide, more often than not it was the *secrecy* that troubled them ... Telling them the truth is the best way to start. Then let them talk as much as possible. Not all families are wonderful, but those who stay around and let the children be involved in their lives give their youngsters a far better chance of a future without depression, or worse.

When death is public news

Many outsiders inevitably become involved when a sudden death becomes a public 'news item'. Imagine seeing the headlines in your local paper: 'Body Found on Railway Line!' Perhaps you can hide that from small children, but what about school friends?

One mother was in court for her husband's inquest. During the evidence it was mentioned that her husband had a row with his son the morning he committed suicide. Spotting a newspaper reporter, the mother asked him to remember that she had three young children. The young man smiled and answered, 'Sorry, lady, it's news.'

Not all reporters are so insensitive, but many children suffer badly in this way – exaggerated headlines, and unnecessary enlargements of photographs can compound the misery. During the early days of bereavement, a child will feel as raw, tender and vulnerable as an adult – perhaps more so – and any careless remark will cause deep pain. A 12-year-old girl overheard her father's suicide being discussed by some bus passengers as though it was an exciting episode in a TV serial. She jumped off the bus and ran home.

An understanding educational psychologist said of such children:

> Totally bereft is an apt description for them ... Their pain is intense, but if I can get in touch with some of their negative feelings and help them to realize that nothing is destroyed by them, that it *is* only their thoughts – then often they begin to cope.

I asked her if it is possible, or wise, to try to help children in such acute distress. Her answer was one I wish all bereaved families could hear:

> If you are a familiar, trusted friend or family member, that's wonderful ... Nothing can be more awful for a child than to be dragged off to a therapist and made to talk about Daddy ... If you are trying to help, especially with children between say, 8 and 14, start by stressing that their feelings are very natural, that none of them are wrong ... They will be feeling insecure ... They need something concrete. What is very important for them to know is that, at some point in time, they were loved by their dead parent. If they are told nothing, they may well believe they were not loved, and therefore think, 'I am bad' – the scar of believing they are not lovable will remain perhaps right into their adulthood. Those are the people we see eventually in therapy. So it's essential that you never try to stop these children talking, even when the tears are falling. I'm sure that not nearly so many young people would come to me carrying burdens of emotional guilt if only someone had listened to them and shared their heartbreak.

Social workers

It is often a social worker who has to gather the various carers in a community together. Both counselling and listening skills are given high priority in their training, and these include techniques to encourage people to talk about the things that are important to them (so vital for rapport among children). Many workers are now attached to hospices and children's hospitals, and liaise with teachers, doctors and local churches. A senior social worker told me:

> We also involve the increasing number of non-professional coun-sellors who are coming forward ... Together we can share our knowledge and experience, and become more self-aware, adapt-able and flexible. This means that we are able to produce a more exciting mix of appropriate help for the bereaved.

Counselling skills for public workers

Listening skills, interpersonal skills and human awareness are now included in police training programmes. Students today are very fortunate. Until very recently our police, fire and ambulance people had to learn from grim experience. 'It's aston-ishing how the public expect us – like doctors and nurses – to be born knowing how to face traumas and cope with disaster,' said one training sergeant. Counselling skills for women police constables include how to deal with rape victims, and they will always be sent into homes where there are children. The police training programme in Surrey, for example, is so comprehensive that many social workers come to the police for guidance in counselling.

In ambulance training, of course, treatment is the main thing. A midwife does come in to give a session on human awareness, but in many areas students receive only a 20-minute talk on bereavement. Less than two decades ago, an ambulance instructor was asked what was covered on bereavement in his training programme and he replied, 'Death and disposal.'

Counselling courses are improving all the time. Students are always accompanied by trained instructors – but in all these pro-fessions death is met fairly quickly and fairly often. No amount of training ever quite prepares any of us for our first struggle to tell sad news, or our first sight of a dead child.

5

The surviving parent

Psychiatrists all say that when one parent dies, the attitude and behaviour of the surviving parent determines that of the children. This is a huge responsibility to add to the heartache of a grieving mother or father. If you want to help bereaved children, start by helping their widowed parent.

When you look at the families where a widow or widower is struggling alone, you find that most of them *are* coping – somehow. Their loss has given them a common purpose and all the members of the family are helping each other. Some flourish, many manage well, most of us muddle through. But it's not an easy task. We've seen how each child in a family can have different reactions, so what the surviving parent does for one may be quite wrong for another.

Trying to cope

Talking with and listening to enlightened experts, as I have, and meeting many widows, widowers and bereaved children has confirmed several of the doubts I've often felt about *my* ability to cope. As a parent, you will have similar doubts. With hindsight, it is easy to see where well-meant help was inadequate, or wrong decisions were taken. But at the time you may well have been too heartbroken to think straight. Or perhaps you were a victim of your own upbringing?

Don't feel guilty. You did what you felt was right at the time. Start from that point, not from your guilt. If you acted through love, that is all that matters, and is what your child will remember.

A young parent's death is usually untimely and sudden, so the surviving partner will be in deep shock, perhaps hysterical, or possibly dry-eyed and numb. Realization of the enforced new role has not yet hit them. The majority are mothers – arguably more able to cope with a young family. But today, when the parental roles are less clearly defined than they used to be, the differences are not so great, certainly in practical terms – a father can change nappies, a mother can run her own business.

For both, a few hours, or even minutes, have changed their lives. A young wife at breakfast is a widow by lunchtime. She has lost her husband, her lover, the father of her children, often her means of financial survival, including, perhaps, her home. Above all, she now has full responsibility for the children.

She will not take all this in at once, and may be without any feelings except for an overwhelming protectiveness towards those children. 'I *can't* tell them their daddy is dead!'

A husband, suddenly left alone with his youngsters, has similar emotions – he's lost the mother of his baby, his beloved wife, the person he shares all his thoughts with, plans the children's future with.

When a mother dies, there is seldom a shortage of surrogate mother figures – a grandmother perhaps, or an aunt – to provide sustenance, care, hugs and cuddles. But when a father dies, it is rare for other men to appear on the scene. A relative or neighbour may provide temporary help for the widow – mow the lawn or fix the car. But what about warm, loving gentleness for daughters and understanding encouragement for sons? There is often no one to fill that enormous void.

Every child's memory of their parent's death is unique – the universal irony being that the only person who might conceivably provide any sort of comfort in this frightening event is the person who has died. The remaining parent has to cope, handle the situation as best he can, knowing that he is *not* the longed-for person.

Insensitive relatives can often hurt by their inability to console a child. 'He's spoiled,' they say, following it up with, 'Don't upset your father.' As though *any*thing a child says or does could upset him more deeply than he is already.

In time children and parents may comfort each other, perhaps draw closer because of their tragedy. But in the immediacy of a sudden death, a parent is often too deeply afflicted to step into the role of comforter. Tiny children will sense the unhappiness without appreciating their parent's sorrow, and become extra demanding. They need the physical closeness and emotional support of their one remaining parent, a reassurance that their world has not entirely collapsed. This is one time when the calm presence of an extended family member or understanding friend will be very welcome.

In your grief, you may never imagine that your children's reactions are very like your own. You think of them as youngsters, very unhappy at losing their father or mother, but not as bereaved people suffering similar grief symptoms.

One widow recalls such a time:

I knew he was dead, yet I called out when I saw a man like him in the street, even ran after him into a shop. Yet it never entered my head that my children might be doing the same thing. How egocentric bereavement can make us.

One teenage girl voiced the memories of many children:

I often walked through the cemetery calling for my dad. I suppose I just wanted to see him. I'd choose to visit my friends' families where the father had the same colour hair, or wore the same type of clothes as my dad.

To ensure the love of their remaining parent, older children tend to hide their emotions, becoming tough throughout the crisis. Only years later, events touching on sensitive areas may reveal their serious wounds caused by those concealed emotions.

Changes in behaviour

Children have to face strange changes in the behaviour of their widowed father or mother. A parent has many ambivalent feelings at this time. One day you want to drive over a cliff, and the next you are terrified to go out in case you have an accident and the children are orphaned.

Parents can become angry and even resent the children. 'I can't even go to the pub to console myself, I have to babysit.' Some are violent towards the baby, or make excessive demands on older children.

Once-loving mothers can become cold and distant, while formerly unemotional women may become extra loving – as if trying to compensate for their years of staying aloof – perhaps taking a child into bed at night. A conscientious father, always home on time, always taking his share of household chores, now cannot face the home without his wife. He stays late at work, goes away for weekends, appears indifferent towards the family – it's his way of coping. Such behaviour changes are usually short-lived, but are very frightening to small children.

A parent's inconsistency can also be bewildering. A distraught widower, filled with his own anxieties, finds it easy to lay blame on a child. One mother, who used to fight constantly with her husband, through her guilt became the traditional inconsolable widow when he died. Her children feel doubly bereaved – this weeping person is not the mother they knew.

Communication between parent and child becomes increasingly difficult. Confidences or responsibilities are sometimes given that a child is not yet capable of taking on.

The whole family will have raw emotions – a tiny hurt can feel like a deep wound. A child may dress in her dead mother's clothes, or pretend to smoke her dead father's pipe; an agonized parent interprets this behaviour as callous and wants to scream at the child to leave the beloved's things alone. One widow was brought up short by her daughter who said, 'You only knew Dad for 14 years, I've known him all my life.' In times of crisis even the behaviour of people you love can so easily be misinterpreted.

On the whole, children are very practical. I asked a family of four boys how their father was coping since their mother had died. 'Fine, he's managing everything OK except the washing machine.'

When children feel guilt

Bobby's father rescued him from drowning, but died hours afterwards from a heart attack. Bobby knows his mother blamed him for the death, and has carried the guilt for several years. Twelve-year-old Annie knows her father had to lose his wife for her to be born – thankfully a rare situation today. Her father adores her, but Annie's feeling of guilt hangs over her.

Some children also feel guilty if they remember things they never liked about their dead parent. But if the surviving parent can discuss their partner with laughter as well as tears, he or she will become not a myth but a parent they can remember as a real person.

Not all families are happy families

Where the home situation is not perfect before a tragedy, sadly a parent's death will probably not change that state of affairs. Perhaps a mother drinks too much, leaves the children alone in the house and returns to knock them about. If her husband dies, she's not suddenly going to turn into a warm-hearted, mother-earth figure.

A father who has never taken any notice of his children may turn to them if his wife dies, find he needs them, and expect them to look after him. Or he may now ignore them completely. It's unlikely he will change into a paragon of fatherhood.

Surviving mothers

'Mum was suddenly sad, always sad. She never, ever, seemed to have a happy face.' 'I never saw my mother cry. I had to go to my grandmother to learn about my father. Mother wouldn't talk about him.' Two conflicting reactions of bereaved young mothers, but both hard for a small child to understand. For however loving a mum is, and many will become more so, she is too shattered to be able to devote all her thoughts to her children in the early days of her bereavement.

Later, the majority of widowed mothers do cope extremely well – especially now that it is not unusual for them to be the breadwinner of the family. If her children are still babies or toddlers, however, this can bring problems. For example, many mothers resent being tied to the house. 'I never thought I'd have to look after them on my own. I feel as if I'm under a life sentence.' It is not an unusual plea, and there is no easy answer.

For some, professional intervention is needed if the family is to survive. Tessa, at 29, is still floundering after two years of widowhood. She is little help to her children of 5, 7 and 8. She never talks to them of their father, never listens to them, but often takes the youngest into her bed and cuddles her. She sees no future, and lethargy is taking over; the tension in her home is enormous.

Fortunately, her doctor has referred Tessa to a clinical psychiatrist, who immediately recognized that Tessa's best hope lies in support from friends or a parent circle. She has no extended family, and feels isolated and afraid. For non-joiners the thought of approaching any group, whether run by a church, school or widows' organization, is daunting. Still too withdrawn to attend herself, Tessa has been persuaded by the psychiatrist to let her children visit a local parent circle with a widowed friend who has a family of the same age group. The children, especially the two older ones, are making friends and being helped to understand they are not 'different' and that their lives *can* carry on as before, once Mum is 'better'.

It will take time, for Tessa still feels that the professional 'can't possibly know how I feel'. But he does understand. He knows how extremely difficult it is for a young mother to care for dependent children when feeling desolate and uncomforted herself. And he also knows he must guard against his patient becoming too dependent upon him for his understanding – she must be encouraged to help herself.

Sadly, 6-year-old Emily's mother never had any counselling help of any kind, and was unable to help her children. The two older ones left home as soon as possible, leaving Emily 'highly embarrassed' by her mother's bouts of weeping in front of her father's photograph. Instead of being taken to friends, or a parent circle, she was sent to boarding school. 'When I visited friends I'd pretend their fathers were mine,' says Emily, 'but I could never bring myself to call them Daddy. Suddenly the word daddy wasn't in my vocabulary any more.'

This lack of loving family support seriously affected Emily's growing up: 'I missed out on a real childhood.' Now in young adulthood she is unable to love anyone for fear of losing them; she cannot even allow herself to keep a puppy or a kitten because 'they might die'.

Sons and daughters without fathers

Ross was in his first year of senior school when his dad died in a road accident. 'Mum can't seem to cope now. She never has a meal ready in the evening. She says she can't afford to buy meat, but there's plenty of whisky in the kitchen.'

For a mother left with sons it can be tough. As they approach puberty she may feel very inadequate. And for boys it is not easy to be left in an all-female household. Some widows acquire an embarrassingly emotional dependency on their sons.

For daughters, father represents adventure, discipline and responsibility, and from him a daughter learns the pleasure of being female. However, loss of a father is not necessarily the road to marital disaster for a girl, as some experts seem to suggest. This must obviously depend on individual circumstances, both before and after the death, and on a girl's relationship with her mother.

Two teenage daughters look back now with gratitude to a mother who kept their dad's memory very much alive:

> Mother couldn't stop talking about Dad after he died, pouring out intimate details of their marriage. I hated it at first. But I realize it's better than a mother who thinks her children can't understand and is not open with them. We cry on Dad's birthday and talk about his work together, and he's still very much part of our family.

Surviving fathers

In the bewildering and bustling aftermath of a young mother's death, all resources will be put towards caring for the children, and very little to the searing feelings of loss of the husband. He seldom has time to grieve.

One young dad was struggling to control his emotions: 'I feel outside reality ... I know I sound selfish, but I can't stop thinking of my wife, she didn't want to leave us. I've got no room inside me, even for my own children.'

For others, the children are their salvation. 'They keep me sane,' says Pete, left with a boy of 3 and a girl of 4. Together they all keep their mother's memory very much alive. Pete made a cake for his daughter's fifth birthday and popped it into the microwave. When it came out very solid, the little girl shook her finger at him. 'Mummy used to put it in the gas oven.'

Two of Mike's children are girls, now nearing puberty. 'I felt so helpless when they were young, I wasn't sure whether to kiss and cuddle them as their mother used to. Now they're older, I feel even more inadequate.'

Girls in an all-male household

It's not always easy if there's only one daughter in the family. Mandy's large, jolly mother died and she was left with a quiet father and two very independent brothers. 'If I was a bit older I could be the mum,' says Mandy, 'but they treat me like a servant.'

Liz lives alone with her father. 'We get on well, but I wish he talked more. He gets upset because I'm growing very like my mother, with the same mannerisms apparently. But I *like* being told that, I was only 10 when she died.'

Surviving parents
after divorce

If the parents were separated before the death of either, the children will have very muddled emotions. If they're living with their mother they tend to blame her for their father's death. If Mum is upset, they wonder why she ever divorced. If she is *not* seen to cry, they accuse her of having no feelings.

A death can increase the bitterness in a separated family. June and Alison were living with their mother when they were told of their father's death in Scotland. To their mother's horror, they accused her of 'letting Dad die – if you hadn't turned him out he'd be alive today!'

Remember that these children have already suffered one major loss. A great deal will depend on how they have adjusted to that separation. Now they have to take on board this new, irreversible loss. They must be encouraged to voice their feelings, questions and worries. How sad when such a family's grief can never be properly shared.

When a parent remarries

From the day her father died, 12-year-old Anthea would keep on asking her mother, 'You're not going to marry again, are you, Mum? There are no nice men like Daddy around.'

Many children have expressed the same immediate reaction to the loss of a parent. The titles of stepmother and stepfather, with their grim traditional overtones of Victorian cruelty, have perhaps added to the natural fears of a child that a strange person will invade their family circle. There is also a very real fear of losing their surviving parent's love – Dad will love her, not me.

Anthea's worst fears were realized when a man friend of her mother's came to stay in the house. 'I shall never forget the day I got up early and found his bed hadn't been slept in. At 14, girls can be very moralistic, and oh, how I created.' She resented this intrusion into the family, and when her mother married the man a year later she refused to attend the wedding.

At its best, such a relationship *can* help to sustain a child. 'I have to show by everything I do or say that I appreciate Sally's attachment to her dead mother,' said one stepmother who is coping well. 'I try to encourage her artistic talents which she inherited from her mother.' It is not an easy role to fill – but for a child such as Liz (see page 51) an understanding wife for her father might well have lessened the tension in their relationship.

Obviously, the age of the children when a parent remarries is significant. During adolescence there will be many nostalgic events or anniversaries, and if one coincides with the arrival of a step-parent, their emotions could be extremely forceful:

Mum died when I was 17. From that day, Dad was out to find another wife. When he did it was disastrous. I hated him and her. I felt I'd lost both parents, because it was never the same. I resented my stepmother, she made me and my brother feel in the way, and never even tried to be nice to us.

Even when the child is very young, even when a new mother or father brings happiness to a bereaved home, it would surely be wrong to expect a child to forget her real parent. No one human being can replace another. Deirdre was only 2 when her widowed father remarried. 'My stepmother was very kind to my sister and me, but we never thought of her as our own mother.'

Christine was 14 when her father died. 'After two years Mum married again. We'd known him a long while, and he never tried to take over as a father figure, he's just a friend. Taking Dad's place? No way! You don't ever replace someone.' Her sister Phillippa, at 12, found it harder – jealousy of someone taking her mother's attention was inevitable. But both sisters were happy that it had not meant leaving their dad's home. That was very important.

Children who have never known one of their parents

The poignant description 'mourning an absence' puts into perspective the ambivalent feelings of children who never knew a dead parent. Most agree they have been aware of a loss – a void in their lives. Amy described it as

> a sort of gap in my life, not a sadness. There were no photos of me with my mother, yet I always felt she was watching me. I'm told the first sentence I wrote in my news book when I started school was, 'My mother is dead.'

Amy feels she has grieved more since growing older, although when she visits her mother's grave she feels nothing except pity for a young woman dying at 27.

Whether or not a child is conscious of being 'deprived' will depend on the surviving parent. One teenage girl whose mother died two days after she was born said, 'I was at school before I realized no one had ever put their arms round me.' A little girl can hardly be more deprived than that.

The danger lies in a child fantasizing her unknown parent. June, whose father died before she was born, is aware of the dangers:

> My mother refused to talk about him, and my fantasies grew enormous. Was I adopted? Was my father still alive? Perhaps he was in prison? I was in my twenties before she told me, on the eve of my own wedding, what a respected member of our neighbourhood he was. Since knowing about him, I've begun to mourn a real person.

In this age of single parents, it becomes even more essential for their children to be given the truth about their births. The truth may be hard to tell and to hear, but it will prevent fantasies and provide trust – vital for successful family lives.

How do bereaved families survive?

Some surviving parents appear, on the surface, to be well controlled. They talk logically, their decisions are rational, their discussions with their children seem full of understanding. Such a widow, or widower, is thought to be so well adjusted that little outside help is offered. 'She's coping,' say neighbours or relatives. I've met widows who show this sort of textbook behaviour, and it is as if they are running on automatic pilot. But what about their children during the flight? Some land safely, others have a fairly bumpy ride, while a few lose control in mid-air.

A close friend can sometimes spot this type of automatic behaviour and guide a parent back to closer communication with his children. A widower was horrified when his brother suggested they go away for a week's climbing. 'I can't leave the children, break their routine; suppose I have an accident? Who will cope?' He was finally persuaded to go and returned exhausted. 'I haven't the energy to get the supper!' he groaned. His 7-year-old daughter flung her arms round him. 'You sound like our real daddy again!' Suddenly, he could talk to his child.

For one mother it took a 10-year-old to bring her down to earth with a bump. 'Why don't you laugh any more, Mum?' was her son's innocent question, and she knew that it was time for her to take her first step towards a 'normal' life again. It cannot be achieved overnight – but if you can help a surviving parent to return to 'manual control' of life, you may be assisting another bereaved family to 'muddle through'.

When both parents die

When children lose both their mother and father, perhaps in a car or plane crash, their grief can hardly be imagined. Natalie's mother died of cancer and the following year her father was drowned. Paul's mother committed suicide after her husband was killed in a terrorist attack. Tragedies abound – and yet extended families, community and church groups, neighbours and friends have all been known to provide the affection and care that is suddenly missing from such children's lives.

Sadly, some families 'slip through the net', as the social workers say. They may be new to a district, be without any close relatives, may simply not belong to any social group or be isolated in a large city. Most parents leave instructions in their wills as to how their material goods should be taken care of, but few nominate a choice of care for their children. It is wise to seek the advice of a solicitor to make decisions legal – sometimes written as well as verbal wishes concerning guardianship are difficult to uphold in law.

'We had no one to turn to'

When children have no extended family able or willing to give them a home, they may find themselves in a children's home or with foster parents. Kathy tells her own story:

> My dad died when I was 8. My brother was 5 and it affected him so deeply I put on a brave face to help him and Mum. I never sat

down and started grieving myself. I kept it inside. I was 14 when Mum was killed by a hit-and-run driver and again I felt responsible for my brother.

Kathy, adult beyond her years, had to contend with the trauma of their family home, which was in the hands of an unscrupulous executor to her mother's will, being sold: 'I wanted to keep it, but he sold it; I don't even know what happened to the furniture.' After a few weeks of being looked after by neighbours, Kathy was sent to a local foster home:

> The worst part was that my brother was sent to the other end of the country. My foster mother obviously only did fostering for the money. I never saw any of the clothing allowance she had for me, but she used to buy videos and washing machines. When it got towards my eighteenth birthday she said she would only be paid up to that date and I'd have to leave. I had nowhere to go, I was really scared; I searched every night for accommodation. I didn't want to live on my own so I went to live with my boyfriend. We're married now. Yes, I've survived but I'm scared to have kids myself in case the same thing happens to them.

Another family, whose parents had been killed in a coach crash, were separated when they were still in primary school: 'My sisters and I felt the authorities were looking for homes for us as though we were stray puppies. For years I thought I was being punished and I didn't know what for.'

No children should have to suffer so much unhappiness on top of their very natural grief at the loss of their parents.

Surviving grandparents

Often it is grandparents who take over, although that is not always the 'cosy' experience it sounds. It is not unknown for both sets of grandparents to put in applications when children are made wards of court, and ugly squabbles can plunge lonely youngsters even deeper into their grief.

It is not an easy task for grandparents. They are an older generation (though they may only be in their late forties or early fifties) and will also be grieving the death of their son or daughter. The old 'survivor's guilt' will be deeply disturbing.

Their grandchildren may be precious to them, and they may love them dearly, but now their lives are going to be tied down again just when they hoped for a bit more leisure time. The children will also feel bitter and bewildered, and guilty when grandpa buys them a new toy.

Granny has a difficult role here. Children of all ages may resent her – she was bearable when she was babysitting, but not now. Granny has to confess she's a permanent substitute. She will feel helpless at first, but hopefully will discover that although her loving care and support won't remove the pain of her little grandchildren, it will help them to bear it.

Where grandparents can help enormously is in keeping alive memories of the parents. 'You're the living image of your mum.' 'Your dad loved music, just like you do.' As time goes by the old family photo albums will be a wonderful tonic. 'Did Daddy have a bike when he was my age?' 'Is that Mum in the netball team?' Children love stories of a parent's childhood, and their remarks, though daunting at times, will help the older generation to keep things in perspective.

6

Death of a sibling

No death appears so poignant as that of a child – a baby in arms, a toddler, a lively schoolchild, or a teenager on the threshold of adulthood. For the parents it's the most painful and least acceptable of any loss. Understandably, sympathy and deep concern pour upon them from all sides. What about their surviving child or children? A loved brother or sister is dead, and everyone is rushing to comfort their mother. Some grown-ups are even saying, 'You must help your mother, dear, she's very upset.'

Aren't children supposed to be upset too? The little brother they helped to feed as a baby and have taken to nursery school every day has died; the big sister they turned to when they needed someone to talk with has suddenly been killed in a bicycle accident; the child they fight and argue with every day but who remains their best friend, and with whom they share a bedroom, isn't ever coming home. Perhaps an only brother has died: 'Now I'm an only child.' They are desolate.

Meanwhile, the parents are far too wrapped up in their own tragedy and may even forget they have other children. They have turned into tearful strangers. A couple whose 10-year-old daughter was killed on a pedestrian crossing were asked how their two teenage sons reacted. 'I've no idea,' said their mother. 'I don't remember even thinking about them.'

For a small child, the death of a parent could be a greater disaster, but the death of a sibling makes him aware of his own mortality. Sometimes a younger child, on reaching the age at which an older sister or brother died, will be very apprehensive.

A loving mother with three sons aged 7, 4 and 2 became shocked into a distant numbness when the youngest boy swallowed a button which choked him to death. She appeared quite unmoved – never spoke of the dead child – and took less instead of more care of the other children, not noticing if they roamed around the neighbourhood, not even shutting the gate onto the road. They grew up believing their mother would not care if they died too.

When there is only one remaining child, this 'shutting away memories' can be cruel indeed.

Guilty distress

When months or years have been spent with a terminally sick child as the focus of the family's attention, the healthy children will have experienced jealousy, pity and anger at their family's sufferings. In bereavement, other feelings will surface – perhaps relief, followed by more guilt. These will show in uncooperative behaviour, either withdrawn or aggressive.

Parents, in their distressed state, may also be angry, and misinterpret this behaviour, or compare it unfavourably with that of the dead child. Distraught mothers have been heard to say, 'You killed her!' recalling a child bouncing on a sick bed or dropping a glass of medicine. Unwisely handled, such experiences cause immense distress, compounding blame with grief and leaving a lifelong sense of misunderstanding and rejection.

Sandy's is a familiar story:

> My parents talk about my brother Leo as if he was some sort of saint – he certainly wasn't. Sometimes when we were playing games he'd cheat, and I'd upset his tray of cards all over his bed and he'd tell me not to be nasty because he was going to die. I thought that was unfair, and I'd be mad at him and take away his pillows. Now I miss him like crazy.

Sandy's mother, however, couldn't understand his unruly behaviour when the adored Leo finally died. 'Why can't you behave like Leo used to?' The more worthless and unloved he felt, the worse Sandy behaved. 'One day I asked Mum if she wished it had been me who had died, and she yelled that of course she did, Leo was a good boy.'

A recent study of such children showed that 'low self-esteem is found to be very common, together with considerable idealization of the dead sibling. For many children, measuring up to the dead sibling seems to be an impossible task.' The chief psychologist at a children's hospital pointed out, however, that a surviving child's self-esteem was related to the length of the patient's illness:

> In general, the longer the illness, the happier the children are with themselves. This may be a reflection of the greater opportunity for parents to adapt to their own forthcoming loss and subsequently help their other children to deal with the experience. High self-esteem is more likely if the child has been told the truth about a fatal illness; participated in the patient's care; been given an opportunity to say goodbye near the time of death; and attended the service or been with family members on the day of the funeral.

A consultant paediatrician spoke of death being 'a family affair' and at a hospice for children I learned what this can mean in terms of brothers and sisters. If the parents are sharing their feelings about the impending death of a sibling, even very young children can stay with a dying child – perhaps hold his hand, or sit beside the bed sharing a picture book.

Toby had leukaemia, and from the day of his diagnosis his younger sister Jane shared his life. She grew accustomed to sleeping in the hospital with her mother; she held Toby's favourite teddy while he had his treatments. It was part of her normal routine. She saw her parents cry when the news was bad, and laughed with them during the times when Toby was well enough to attend school. Her grief was huge when he died but she was able to express it *with* her parents. Families such as Toby's and Jane's *are* coping. They have grown in togetherness.

If they have become used to visiting, children are encouraged to see the dead body, and this always seems to help allay fears and fantasies that half-truths can cause. Even following an accident, the reality is often far less traumatic than the visualizations of a young imagination. One child of 6 showed no emotion at seeing her dead sister, and some hours later calmly told me she thought when you died your head went to heaven. 'You said only the body would be left,' she said. Another child took that even more literally, understanding a 'body' to mean simply a torso. 'He's left his arms and legs!'

But those who do see the body are glad they did. Even children like Miles, who was 9 when his 7-year-old sister died of cancer. Now, 13 years later, he talks of it as vividly as if it was yesterday. 'I was allowed to spend time with her on my own. She looked healthier than she had for ages, but it was just a carcass, no longer human.' Yet Miles treasures that memory 'as the most secure and private part of me, something that strengthens me because I know that nothing life can bring will be worse than that'.

When a sibling commits suicide

Children whose brother or sister commits suicide could, understandably, challenge Miles's remark. They are overwhelmed with emotions – often starting with guilt. 'Did we quarrel?' 'Was I so horrid to live with?' They feel anger too. 'How could he have upset Mum and Dad so much?'

There is also a confusing jealousy, because there's romance attached to suicide, a sort of Romeo and Juliet drama. The dead sibling becomes a martyr: look at all the attention he's getting after committing the act.

Meanwhile, their parents will be suffering the searing agony of imagined failure alongside their heartbreak, and may be too devastated to notice their other children. Patricia remembers when her brother killed himself after failing his exams. 'I don't think Mum knew how much I cried, or if I came in for meals, or even slept at home. If my aunt had not come and taken me away I think I might have killed myself too – just to get Mum's attention.'

Thank goodness for all the relatives, friends and good neighbours who *do* step in on such occasions. It's one time when 'looking in on next door' is *not* an intrusion, when 'taking over' is *not* interfering; it's essential, often life-saving.

If you can't cope, or feel the children are too distressed to accept your help – don't hesitate to call your doctor or ask for a counsellor. Often it may be necessary to contact several sources before a satisfactory approach for those particular children is found. A psychiatric consultant confirmed this view:

> All sorts of reasons are often given for psychiatrists *not* getting involved. Often a teacher feels unable to discuss death; a parent won't admit his inability to help his own child; an older brother or sister says it's too sensitive a subject to take outside the family.

But the consultant genuinely wants to help prevent difficulties later on. 'What matters most is that between them, all the carers involved prove to the young bereaved family that loving support is at hand, that their surviving parents *will* become themselves again, and that somebody cares.'

'Someone was thinking about me'

Mark is 30 now, a successful lawyer. Fifteen years ago, when he was a rebellious teenager, 'thoroughly unlovable' (his words), his elder brother overdosed after a sad love affair. Mark's parents collapsed; his father took to drink and his mother had to be hospitalized:

> A neighbour came in and took me for a long walk on the Downs. I was mad, real mad, and wanted to hit him, but he was a big man,

a footballer. We must have walked for hours, and he took me back to his house and his wife gave me a huge meal. Then we watched TV and they came and sat either side of me and each took a hand and held it tight. That meant more to me than any words. I didn't become an 'easy' teenager overnight, but from that moment I knew that someone was thinking about me.

Funerals

Families dread the day – it looms as an enormous hurdle that has to be 'got over' somehow. Following a sudden death, shock may prevent any hope of the family being able to make their own arrangements. But if the team of carers who have known their child in his illness continues to guide them through the period after the death, parents often find comfort in preparing their child's service. If they are old enough, brothers and sisters can help to choose flowers and music; 7-year-old Toby's school friends made little posies and came to the church. The little white coffin, though heartbreakingly poignant, seemed to symbolize a hope of spring. Quite different from a girl who recalls her sister's funeral in the 1930s when 'it was dark and cold in church and everyone seemed to be red and blotchy'.

The traditional 'coming back to the house for tea' is a tough time. A child will long for the talkative relatives and strange grown-ups to go away. And the realization that the dead sister is not there to help her, or to slip upstairs and giggle with, can suddenly hurt unbearably.

The lonely weeks ahead

One boy spoke of the whole crisis as a 'make or break time' for families, and in the lonely weeks and months to come this is strikingly true. On the whole, families deal with death as they deal with life. How sad when a child is thwarted in her efforts to 'get back to normal'. A young teenager sobbed uncontrollably when talking about an interfering neighbour:

> Just because I went to a disco with my friends the week after my brother's funeral, she stopped me and asked, 'How could you? With your brother hardly cold in his grave?' I hated her more than I've ever hated anyone in my life. How could she know how much I miss my brother?

Sometimes even the immediate family, blinded by their sorrow, can be similarly hurtful to each other.

Mary, at 13, loved talking about her older sister who died after a short illness. 'Can I go to France like Rosie did?' But every mention of Rosie's name started Mum crying, and finally Mary kept quiet, spending the evenings in her room playing her sister's old records. 'My parents obviously wanted to be alone. With Rosie gone, I had no one to pour it all out to.' She never showed any aggression at home, but after being sick at school one day, she began to pour out her thoughts to the school nurse, telling her that she was scared of the 'violent feelings' she sometimes had towards her mother. On being told, her mother appreciated that she was not helping her lonely daughter. But she still finds it almost impossible to climb out of her own heartbreak.

Sometimes, as time goes by, parents channel all their ambitions into one such remaining child – and the expectations becoming dauntingly high. Children try to become like a dead sibling, and begin to lose their own identities.

Death of a handicapped child

Another cause of guilty distress can be the death of a sibling who is physically or mentally handicapped. It may, in the case of congenital disease, have been expected – but when a family's life has centred round this special child for so many years, probably with an enormous amount of loving care, the surviving children may worry about unexpected feelings of relief that creep over them. They know their lives will change: they won't now have to push the wheelchair instead of cycling to school; they can have friends to the house without the embarrassment of a sometimes uncontrollable brother or sister; they hope to enjoy more of their parents' attention.

They will also feel a huge void in their lives, and find they are mourning, as deeply as their parents, for a 'might have been', for a brother who *might* have played football with them but never could.

Those outside the family circle find it hard to understand and cope with the reactions of the siblings. Responses such as 'Now I can have his bed,' and 'We can go on holiday this year,' make children of all ages sound uncaring and impervious to loss.

The headmistress of a special school, with wide experience of handicapped children and their families, says that the greatest help for these bereaved children comes from other families:

> There is a tremendous bond among them. There are also very close relationships within these families, for in order for them to function successfully, each person has had an important part to play – they work as a team – their lives have been geared to that child's needs since the day he was born.

She also added that when a handicapped child dies, 'the family has not only lost a child, but financial assistance also. Siblings are left worrying about a future with less money.' (In the UK a large number of allowances and benefits are administered by the Department for Work and Pensions (DWP) specifically for handicapped people.)

A public tragedy

Bereavement can be a hugely isolating state – no other situation can make you feel more truly alone. However, when there is a public disaster – a coach, plane or train accident, a fire tragedy or a horrific terrorist attack – there *is* more support. Communities rally round, and strangers as well as neighbours often provide overwhelming help.

But sometimes such help lasts only as long as the headlines, and the future years can be doubly lonely. In Aberfan, for example, the little village in Wales where 116 children died in one morning in 1966 when their school was buried beneath a collapsed coal waste tip, there are any number of tragic stories still being enacted 40 years later.

Many of the mothers still weep daily for their lost children; others have been dry-eyed ever since – old photographs and clothes all destroyed, denying their little child ever existed. As if their own sorrow at losing brothers and sisters and school friends was not enough, the children who survived have had little chance to complete their grieving in such devastated, insecure homes. One father has never worked since his son died in that catastrophe. His 9-year-old daughter was saved, but she has grown up feeling *her* life is worth nothing. She has been bereaved not only of a brother, but of a once-loving father.

Stillbirth

Again, all sympathies after a stillbirth will be directed at the mother – it is a heartrending disappointment: *your* baby, and he's never been alive in your arms.

But hopefully someone, a relative or friend, will remember the small brother or sister waiting excitedly at home for the new arrival. The nursery will be ready, the cot clean and shining, and now there's no baby to put inside it. Instead of their happy mum coming home from the hospital, there's a sad, withdrawn person who hugs them but doesn't seem to be listening when they talk. They are very unhappy, and can be left with a fear of broken promises, and possible fantasies that only an understanding relative or close family friend can help to dispel.

In the past, a stillborn or neonatal baby was 'disposed of' quickly. Today, doctors appreciate that a mother's natural sorrow is more easily expressed when she has a chance to see and hold her dead baby. Many hospitals encourage the whole family to be present – the idea being that children will have something tangible to mourn, not an unidentified lump in Mummy's tummy. They also enable children to see the baby's body in its casket, to put toys in beside it, and of course attend the funeral.

I feel this is a very personal decision for each family. It is different from seeing a child who they have known, lived and played with – such as Toby (see page 60). Some small children might *not* be left with easy memories. 'She's cold, Mummy, she doesn't move.' (It is quite usual to have photographs taken of the baby, which might provide happier memories for some families; but again, this is an entirely optional suggestion.)

Cot death

Even more devastating is the healthy, much-loved baby who one day stops living. A 6-year-old ran into my class one morning and in a loud voice announced, 'My baby's dead and Mummy's screaming!' No tears, but highly charged excitement – and a very disruptive member of the class for many weeks. The loving parents, an older sister and supportive friends all showed great patience, although his grandmother asked me if I thought he was showing off. 'Andy doesn't seem to care,' she said. 'Can a 6-year-old feel grief?'

A few months later he came in and stood by my desk. 'Our baby would have had his first birthday today,' he said, almost nonchalantly. Then he seemed to consider the matter and looked to see if I was still listening. 'I cried at breakfast,' he added. He stayed very close all morning as we read and painted and sang our nursery rhymes. Yes, I was able to tell his granny, little boys of 6 *can* feel deep grief.

Another little boy, only 5, also very active and often naughty, resented his baby sister, was jealous of her, and frequently asked his mother: 'Why can't you take her back to the hospital?' When she died one night he became silent. He felt his behaviour had caused her death, it was all his fault.

To compound the sorrow, such deaths frequently involve legal ramifications, and neighbours can become suspicious rather than sensitive. They have been known to put subtle questions to the other children. 'Did Mummy ever leave Patrick alone with you, dear?' Children sense that suspicion even if they don't understand the implications. Mystery is added to their shock and sadness. A consultant paediatrician writes:

> It is all too easy for those who should be offering support to be pointing fingers. It may be the task of a perceptive friend of the family to suspect and help this kind of trouble, as parents may be too self-absorbed at such a time to notice.

So how does he suggest friends can help?

> The first essential is a willingness to be involved in someone else's grief – an involvement which is bound to be emotionally costly. Remember that upholding parents is a direct means of helping their children. Try to keep the family together in their grief. Children must see everyone cry. Then, as the days go by, make sure they all have some happy outings, play times, even short holidays with friends. It will bring them all closer together.

If she is still young, the mother will often have another baby. Excitement can be tinged with ambivalent emotions. 'Doesn't Mummy like *us*?' 'Will the new baby die in his cot?' Yet bereaved families cope amazingly well and the new baby can be a tonic for all of them. Often it is relatives or friends, with their suggestions of the baby being a 'substitute', who show a lack of understanding and can alienate the other children.

Memories

Anniversaries cannot be avoided. Children will remember a brother's birthday, a sister's funeral date. An empty place will continue to be noticed at the Christmas table.

'I remember buying six pantomime tickets through habit,' said one young father. 'I still think of us as a family of six, not five.' I've heard such actions described as 'macabre' by those who have never known bereavement – but they can be healthy signs within happy families who are, as young Miles put it, 'living with one member of the family absent'. Their strength lies in talking about the absent member, keeping their memory very much alive; we must all learn to respect each other's ways of grieving, of coping.

Young children are very resilient, but they need encouragement. After her brother died Jane, aged 5, asked her mother, 'Can I have Toby's room now?' Another child wanted her dead sister's toys. It's a confusion of jealousy and of not wanting to 'let go' of the lost sibling – a healthy mixture of emotions, so long as a parent is understanding and courageous enough to accept their ideas with a smile. 'Of course, Toby would want you to be in his room,' or 'Yes, I hoped you would look after Jill's toys for her.' It is very tough on the parents, but inside that child will be a huge unspoken gratitude that approval has been given of their way of handling this crisis.

Divided families

There are other, far more tragic families, where perhaps the grieving of the father and the mother take very different paths – paths that can never meet – and the family is torn apart rather than brought closer together by its sorrow. So the surviving children have to take on board yet another loss, of a supportive home. Conversely, a family may have been divided long *before* one child dies, and added distress will follow as the separated parents both visit the sick child and attend the funeral. There may be bitter accusations. 'Why did you let him travel alone?' 'Why didn't you get another specialist to see her?'

There may be demands to take over custody of the surviving children 'as consolation', or sometimes emotional fights or arguments with step-parents or grandparents.

'My sister has died. Isn't that enough tragedy for one family? Do they have to fight as well?' This anguished cry from a boy of only 15.

Trying to understand a child's feelings

A nursing sister, with years of experience among dying children and their families, still spoke humbly when I asked for her advice:

> Those who have themselves experienced a similar type of bereavement can help as no one else can. I cannot say to a little boy whose brother has died, 'I understand how you feel, dear.' I don't. I simply try to get across that I *care* how he feels, and *do* understand that whatever he does or says just now is completely acceptable. Once children trust you they will talk, perhaps release some private worries.

7

School attitudes

'I think my teachers realized they didn't know how to cope.'

Liz spoke of a generation ago, but many teachers still feel inadequate when it comes to coping with bereaved children. This is sad, because schools and teachers can play a vital part in helping youngsters come safely through their grieving. After all, except for the holidays, school makes up quite a large part of each day. After any tragedy, a familiar daily routine can be supportive, comforting, and safe.

It can even provide a feeling of relief. Patsy, left with her elderly, obsessively grieving father, said, 'I used to go to school for laughs, as a sort of entertainment compared with the serious atmosphere of home.'

Conversely, some children become very reluctant and anxious about going to school. There are many reasons for this. Initially, it may well be because children expect their parents to keep them safe, and the loss of either one leaves them feeling vulnerable, anxious and depressed. A great deal of this anxiety centres round the safety of the surviving parent. Barbara was a bright little 8-year-old, but cried each time her mother left her at school. She seemed to recover by mid-morning, then by the afternoon she was anxious and sometimes too tearful to work. She was afraid her mother might get ill or die, just as one day the previous term her father had died while she was at school.

Returning to school

It is usually recommended that children should return to school as soon as possible after the funeral. However, it is vital that cooperation exists between teachers and parents on the right time for the return. As with so many decisions, it is a very individual one.

'You need me,' Neil sobbed to his father, and clung to him when he tried to leave him at his primary school – a heart-rending and yet fully understandable cry from a sensitive 9-year-old who felt he was wanted at home after the death of his mother. Wisely, the head teacher realized the child *had* to be allowed to go home and do what he felt was right. It took time for Neil to be reassured that his father was well and not going to die.

Returning to school can be difficult. Facing your teacher and your friends takes a good deal of courage – wondering whether they know, or understand, what you have been through. As all bereaved people know, well-meaning acquaintances make astonishingly hurtful remarks. However, although insensitive in other ways, children have a more natural and kindly attitude towards their bereaved friends than some adults have towards the bereaved parents. How many times in recent years have we seen schoolchildren hugging their friends who have suffered a tragedy – often openly crying with them.

But teachers must at all times watch for teasing or bullying. Matthew became aggressive for a whole term after his father died; he resented all adults and anyone in authority, seldom smiled at school, his natural gregariousness turned to sullenness towards his friends. One day he told his mother that his best friend had yelled, 'I bet your dad died just to get away from you.'

When a surviving parent is under too much stress to be sufficiently in touch with his own child's needs, teachers who have an ongoing contact with their pupils are often the first to notice symptoms of disturbance.

A teacher's most important job, however, is not to wait for a tragedy to occur – bereavement is not the best time for an objective study of death and its consequences – but to talk with children about death whenever the opportunity arises. It is the best way to counteract the taboo that leads to built-in repression of curiosity and all sorts of irrational fears and nightmares. To be able to meet such a task in a relaxed way, teachers, particularly of senior pupils, need sanction and support. At one university a student teacher's planned thesis on 'How to talk to children about death' was turned down as 'not educational'.

Many teachers are ambivalent about how deeply they should get involved; 'Children need to be protected from such subjects,' is a comment still heard in some staffrooms. Others tend to anticipate problems. Sue, whose daughter was due to start at her first school the term after her father was killed, was told that young Sarah would be put in the problem class, 'because obviously she will be a problem child'. That headmistress had never met the little girl and sensibly Sue entered her for another school in the area.

At senior level also, a bereaved child is sometimes *expected* to be 'different'. An intelligent 15-year-old said:

> The biggest problem at school was my reports ... From the term that Mum died until I left school, every report said, 'Considering the stress that Elizabeth has been under, her work has been exceptionally good.' It was always given as a way out.

There is also a danger of bereaved children being grouped together with other 'one-parent' families – a particularly hurtful expression for widows or widowers – causing teachers not to appreciate the specific needs of a newly bereaved child.

Awareness of these needs is now growing within the caring professions. Let's hope it will extend into the classroom, so that children such as Annette will not be subjected to the ignorance she suffered when only 10 years old. Four weeks after her mother died, her class teacher told the grieving father, 'Your daughter is perfectly readjusted now, she just needs pushing ...'

Courses in bereavement counselling

Even in the 1990s, many teachers were still leaving college without having been offered any guidelines on bereavement counselling. Teacher training colleges I have visited vary in their pastoral curricula. Some offer short optional courses on 'adolescent counselling'; one included a lecture with the ambiguous title of 'Death in the Classroom'; only one listed the subject of 'handling of bereavement'.

Given that the aim of the 'pastoral' teaching in senior schools is to build up young people's social competence, understanding and resources so that they can cope with life's problems as they arise – why do teachers not select subjects such as death and mourning? At college they now study counselling skills such as communication, listening, health and hygiene and personal interests, which could appropriately underlie the caring, concern and empathy vital for bereavement care. The trouble is that in large schools the range of pastoral subjects is *so* wide that, as one educationist put it, 'those on bereavement do tend to get overlooked'.

Organizations such as Cruse Bereavement Care run courses specifically for teachers on helping with bereaved children. But when 250 schools received invitations to a course in the south of England, only 35 teachers attended. 'Quite unnecessary, anyone can comfort a child,' was one comment, while other teachers protested that 'It's a job for the clergy.' It appears it is not easy to keep the balance right.

At all levels of education there are some teachers who are naturally more able to handle the many unexpected crises that occur in any school or college. One sixth-form pupil said, 'It's curious, but after our sessions on death, at the end of the term I felt I understood more about life.' Her teacher had obviously got it right.

There is now far more literature on the subject available to all schools – there are packs and guides on the subject at all levels (see Useful addresses and Further reading). These are not written as formal lessons, but as suggested resources for teachers wanting to help their pupils explore feelings of loss and grief. At the time of writing, a small group in the south of England is putting together a pack for schools to coincide with the creation of a garden of remembrance for children. Let's hope others throughout the UK will come up with similar ideas.

Primary school

In the lower half of a primary school a teacher is almost a mother to the children in her care. She is in an ideal position to listen to their troubles and spot their disturbances. In fact, it is often a teacher who notices a child's unusual behaviour or anxiety before a parent – especially if that parent is in trouble herself.

But long before a tragedy occurs, it does no harm to talk about such 'taboo' subjects as stealing, lying, illness, hospitals and death. Bringing them in casually so that the children quickly come to know that their teacher can be approached on any subject is the best idea. If a teacher appears diffident – and children soon sense if an adult is not willing to talk – then when a crisis happens and a child wants to ask questions or express a worry, he will not have anyone to turn to.

One understanding head teacher has a school in a busy suburb, and she and her staff are of invaluable help to families, especially to a remaining parent with an only child. Jake, with no siblings to turn to and feeling very alone with his grieving father, appeared to be recovering well from his mother's death; he had come through many 'stages' of bereavement, including furious anger with his father, resentment of his teacher, and also a long period of withdrawal. Then his dog was run over, and many of the symptoms reappeared. His class teacher appreciated that this latest trauma had reopened emotional wounds, and together with the school doctor gave young Jake the support he needed.

That head teacher says, 'A teacher must watch for a child's maturity to catch up with her experience, and help her towards it.' One 10-year-old bereaved pupil became withdrawn and unable to concentrate, her school work suffering as a result. The teacher assured her that this was normal, that it was nature's way of giving her a rest until she was strong enough to take the strain of her sadness. 'We had to judge when the time had come to ease her out of herself again.' The ethos in that school is one of total honesty and adult availability for questions, comfort, security and love.

By the time a child leaves his primary school, his teachers should have ensured that he is able to talk naturally of death as 'part of life'. Alert teachers should recognize the many opportunities that offer themselves, even in an inner-city classroom. Perhaps the easiest and most obvious of all are the four seasons and the annual cycle of life and death.

In one city school they kept a pet rabbit. When it died, the head teacher wanted it taken away overnight, but one young teacher insisted the children see it, place it in a box and bury it – not with great ceremony but very simply during their break period. They found a place under a tree in the playground, and the next day children brought plants to make a garden round the grave. They also started to make a book about the rabbit, with photographs, drawings or paintings, and the teacher suggested they write its life story. It made a beautiful book and quietly, without emphasis, more lessons were learned – happy memories should be kept alive and talking about a sad loss makes it easier to accept.

Suggestions for a primary teacher's 'bereavement notebook'

Remember that each child is an individual. Several caring organizations now issue leaflets giving guidelines to teachers, or hold courses on counselling. The message that comes across loud and clear in them all is: 'Take cues from the child's behaviour.'

My own list, compiled from talking with many professionals, teachers and children, all of whose experiences have greatly widened my own, will perhaps serve as a start for a teacher's own notebook.

1 Watch for changes in behaviour

Withdrawal, aggressiveness, anger, nervousness, sullen moods, and lack of concentration are likely within the first few weeks. Handle them with patience, never show that you are surprised or disconcerted. Never be cross.

2 When a child wants to talk, find time to listen

In a class of busy, energetic and demanding children this is not easy. Take the child to one side, explain that you would like to talk, and name a quiet time when you can do so. When the time comes, listen not only with your ears, but with your eyes and your heart.

Cuddle her or, if she seems reluctant, hold her hand. Touch can be reassuring for someone who has lost a warm, loving parent, it lets a child know that you *care*, that you will be there any time they need help.

Encourage them to speak of their parent, and do so yourself. 'I needed to talk about Mum and it was hard with my friends,' said a normally gregarious little boy.

3 Try to involve a child's special friends

If you can gather some 'best friends' in your little talks, show them that when someone you love dies it is good to keep all the happy memories alive by talking about them.

4 Be ready for questions and always be honest

A child often becomes burningly curious about death and burial. A teacher should never be afraid to say 'I don't know.' It is vitally important to find out the family's cultural background and religious views. For whatever your own feelings, they must never conflict with those of the parent, or confuse a young child.

5 Show children it is not shameful to cry

If your eyes fill with tears, if other children join you, let them. Mummy was precious, of course we are sad. Keep a balance by having many light-hearted stories during this time also. Demonstrate that it is possible, and permissible, to smile and laugh. 'Mummy loved clowns, didn't she?' may start a chat about the circus, and drawing time that morning could include painting the big top.

6 Never say, 'You don't mean that, do you?'

Don't say this hoping to allay a child's fears, or trying to change the subject. When Roger said he thought he had caused his father's death, he meant it. Children are honest, they say what they mean. Feelings are real, strong sensations which must be acknowledged, believed and discussed.

Also don't be tempted to say, 'You'll soon feel better.' Far better to say, 'I know how you feel and we don't understand why your daddy had to die so young. We only know that he loved you and that you'll never, ever, forget him.'

7 Try to keep in close touch with the surviving parent

A child will quickly sense if there is a rapport between you and her family, and if it is genuine this will give her added comfort and security. With the cooperation of your head teacher, discuss with the parent any behavioural changes at home, and compare notes on habits such as eating and sleeping.

Teachers should also be sensitive to special days or occasions that may be difficult for bereaved children. Obvious examples would be Mother's Day or Father's Day, when one happy idea would be to find out if a child without a mother has a granny for whom they can make a Mother's Day card. Here again, a teacher must take cues from the child.

It is impossible to be sensitive to every occasion. I heard a teacher reprimanding a girl for refusing to go on a nature walk. Later we discovered that the walk took them past the local fire station, and her father had been a fireman, killed in a rescue attempt earlier that year. No one can be protected from everything; it isn't possible, or healthy. Part of the learning process is to accept that life is not always easy, or fair. We all need some adverse experiences to toughen us ready for the next challenge.

With an understanding teacher in the background, and armed with the knowledge that death is *not* a taboo subject, a bereaved child will have a far better chance of coming through her grief without prolonged or lasting difficulties. Of course, some children whose school work or behaviour continue to give cause for concern will need referral to the school nurse and perhaps a child guidance clinic. Experts agree that such referrals deserve priority in this age group. In some cases, specialized individual psychotherapy may be indicated for child and parent, and often family therapy may be helpful.

Secondary schools

The years between the ages of 11 and 18 are times of great change. A child has many decisions to make. Which exam subjects to take? Should I go on to further education?

There is physical change also as children grow from childhood into adulthood. That means more decisions to be faced. When should they start going out with members of the opposite sex? How late should they be allowed to stay out at night? How do you balance time for homework with work in the house, with television, with sleepovers with friends? Having only one parent to discuss these problems with can mean that teenagers often don't discuss them at all, or blurt them out in an embarrassed fashion and so receive equally unbalanced answers. At this level, young people have very strong views on many subjects, and are beginning to question those of adults in authority. Many have assumed a 'don't care' attitude to several major issues. All mothers know the 'So what?' answer to their dire warnings of the short life of motorcyclists or the importance of acquiring some reasonable exam results.

In the same way that 'having a baby' merely encompasses a pregnancy and possibly a small bundle in a carrycot, with no thought for the two decades of responsibility to follow, so 'dying' means a hospital and a funeral, with no thought for a lifetime of deprivation and loss – *until it happens in your family.* It is particularly sad if a bereavement occurs before any preliminary discussions on death have taken place in the classroom.

Death as a classroom topic

Children today face subjects unheard of a generation ago. Schools arrange lectures and discussions on drug and alcohol abuse, contraception and abnormal sex practices, childbirth and its possible complications, abortion, infertility and surrogate motherhood. Subjects such as paedophilia are openly discussed among pupils of all ages, and often children write theses on mugging and violence in our society – most of these subjects involve pain or illness, or even death. Yet death as a classroom subject is still rare.

Why? It is a human experience which will touch all of us at some time. Doctors, psychiatrists and counsellors stress that learning about death – considering its consequences and realizing its inevitability – is a necessary part of education as a preparation for life and a contribution to psychological growth.

It is, naturally, a very emotive issue for teenagers, which teachers should approach with sensitivity and feeling. In the UK, a teen pack containing guidelines for adolescents, with notes for teachers and counsellors, has been researched and published by Cruse Bereavement Care (see page 113).

It is a huge responsibility for teachers, and a good head teacher will ensure it is shared among the most appropriate members of his staff – he cannot assume that the physics, religious education or biology teacher will take on the subject alone. Some schools involve parents and visiting counsellors.

A good introduction would be to discuss causes of death – old age, illness, violence, including accidents, murder and suicide. This may lead to talking about registering deaths, or hospitals and hospices. Death and obituary columns in a local newspaper can be studied. A child may ask, 'What is an undertaker's job apart from driving a hearse and carrying a coffin?'

Weekly discussions could include questions about priests, burials and cremations. 'Has anyone visited a cemetery?' Visits could be arranged, and a teacher can point out historical, famous or amusing headstones. Different cultures and religions will emerge, and it would be a happy idea to encourage children to learn of the varying funeral rituals and mourning customs from each other. Secular funerals can also be discussed (see page 93).

From now on, discussion periods may become more personal, and a teacher has to assess whether all pupils wish to take part. Usually, they all want to listen, even if they don't speak.

Learning how to comfort bereaved friends

'How to give help and comfort to someone who is bereaved' could be a subject thrown open for general discussion. You might ask if this is necessary. Public tragedies, such as motorway pile-ups or senseless killings of innocent victims, too often appear on our television screens. And these are always followed by heartbreaking scenes of families and friends comforting each other; and have you noticed that by far the most demonstrative are the young people – often schoolchildren – hugging and crying together? With their sharing of tears, and offerings of flowers, surely they know all about the art of comforting? Certainly their outpourings of love and support are a wonderful start – but it is interesting to note that as the days go by very few suggest *talking* about the dead relative. And it is difficult to explain the strong desire, almost longing, that a bereaved person has to talk of their loved one.

'If you died, would you like us never to mention you again?' a teacher asked a cynical teenager. Getting no response, he mentioned John Lennon. 'The day he was shot, suppose we'd all kept quiet? No photos of him, no records played, what would his widow and child have felt?' Suddenly, with this example, her class saw the vital necessity of keeping memories alive.

Teachers (and parents) should always be alert to classmates' reactions when a child dies, especially their close friends; or if a child's lifelong friend from his street dies. The emotional depths of grief suffered can be similar to those of a bereaved sibling.

When it comes to grief, teachers have to remember they are talking to adolescents. In times of stress, some teenagers revert to childhood and communicate with actions rather than words. Andrew's mother died of cancer when he was 15. He was always the quiet one of his school 'gang'. Now he became noisy, a show-off in class, violent towards his friends, and insolent to his teachers. Through discussions with the head teacher and a school counsellor, Andrew's friends had their first lesson on grieving. Andrew's anger and guilt were explained. It took time – and his friends tried to help, although they often ended up fighting. But it made them think about death and what it would mean to them, even what it would mean to die. The reality was a long way from the 'Bang, bang, you're dead!' games they used to play.

As an accompaniment to such discussions, teachers could provide lists of relevant books to read, both fiction and non-fiction (see Further reading).

When a child in the school suffers a major loss, the head teacher can create the atmosphere of 'teacher availability' so essential for pupils in need of support. One head teacher showed me his list of preparations he considers vital if a school is to be of genuine help to a family:

1 When a child first enters the school, teachers must be informed of any previous bereavements, and the class teacher must tell the child that he knows, without making him feel 'different'.

2 The school should provide a suitable, unoccupied room where a child can come at any time he needs a bolt-hole if overcome with tears, or wants to be alone.

3 A bereaved child must be included as part of his peer group.

4 Sometimes an older child needs to be allocated as a confidante – perhaps one with a similar experience for support when necessary.

5 The parents and the rest of the family will also need support; it is vital to know the parents' beliefs, and how much they have told the child.

6 Teachers can help bereaved families on special school days such as parent evenings, speech days, etc.

That school list contains sound advice. We've seen how children tend to 'hold back', afraid to upset the remaining parent, either by crying or causing the parent to cry. It can be therapeutic for a child to talk with a teacher who is willing to listen.

'I quarrelled with my father,' said Pete, weighed down with guilt and unable to tell his mother. His teacher had repeatedly to assure him that everyone quarrels, it's natural, and that his father would not wish him to feel guilty. Kate was upset because her father had bought her grey socks instead of the regulation white for gym, and said she missed her mother 'to go shopping with'. It was necessary for her teacher to appreciate the serious-ness of Kate's worry – hers was a real cry for help, just as much as Pete's.

Although teachers today attend seminars on counselling, some still feel inadequate and are tempted to refer a child they feel to be 'difficult' to an educational psychologist. When is such a step necessary? An experienced social worker said, 'A father's death does not make his child a patient,' and went on to advise that referrals should only be made after joint consultations with the parent, doctor, head teacher and school nurse.

Practical ways to help concentration in bereaved teenagers

A child may appear deep in thought and lose all concentration during these early days. However annoying it may be when they forget what you've asked or told them, try to be patient, quietly repeat your request, or tell them you also forget things.

Their work may deteriorate to such an extent that they need to repeat a term or more of study, especially if exam time is approaching. Literary subjects, demanding creative thought, pose particular difficulties. Telling a child to try harder, or stop daydreaming, does little good. She will be mentally disorganized, so suggest she approaches her work as she does her favourite sport. Betty tried this:

> Before each maths lesson, I pretended I was at the swimming pool. I talked to myself like an athlete, told myself to breathe correctly, imagined I was poised on the edge of the pool before a race. I almost heard the starter gun going off, and when the maths lesson began I really think my mind stopped wandering.

Such a method will not hasten the grief process, but it sometimes allows a pupil to keep her mind on her work enough to keep up with her class.

The cause of deteriorating work is not always obvious. Tara, nearly 17, came from a large family. She was bright, expected to go to college. Then her mother died and her work suffered drastically. When this continued into the following term, her teacher got Tara to talk about it. 'I have to stay up until one in the morning doing the books for my father's business. My mother always did them. It's tiring after doing the housework and cooking for my little brothers.'

The class teacher spoke to Tara's father, who at first resented the school's interference. But once he understood that their only concern was that Tara should go to university, he found someone else to help him, and Tara graduated with success.

The same teacher pointed out that sometimes it is necessary to make children conform, when they use bereavement as an excuse for poor work. 'You have to be sensitive to know when a child is doing just that. After all, as with adults, it is far better for a child to be kept busy.'

Those who criticize young people today don't always appreciate the growing number of moral, social and health behaviour choices they have to face. A glance at the 'pastoral' curriculum of a senior school will surprise many parents. Teachers do a great deal to help our children formulate their maturing attitudes to life. Hopefully, more of them will soon extend that help to include 'consideration of death and its consequences' as part of the official curriculum.

8

Religious attitudes

'Bereavement releases an awful lot of love in a family.'

Hearing a Church of England chaplain say those words gave me great hope in the comfort and support a religious faith can give to a bereaved family. His was the voice of compassion. He knows that grief is the price we pay for love: the greater the love the deeper the sorrow.

This seems to me the role that religion can play today – providing sincere yet uncritical understanding, while appreciating that families differ in their beliefs. In the UK, many children still attend Sunday schools and have Bible stories read to them; they are taken to occasional church services by their parents, but have no rigid rules or beliefs instilled into them. The choice, as with political affiliations, is theirs; and living as we do in a multicultural society that choice is a wide one.

The days are gone when everyone appeared to believe in God without questioning; in the Christian churches, this meant believing in a life 'hereafter'. Small children usually take readily to this idea of life after death, if only because they cannot imagine being 'nowhere'. Most of them happily accept the concept of heaven, although the idea of it being a reward for good behaviour while on earth has thankfully fallen away since Victorian times. Today, a tiny child can be quietly comforted by imagining a precious parent being in a 'happy place' rather than in a hole underground.

We've seen, however, how trite and misguided explanations of death can damage a child's faith and trust, causing fear, confusion and nightmares. It is, of course, as difficult for ministers of religion as it is for anyone confronted with a bereaved family to know what to say. Sadly, many still use old-fashioned, clumsy words.

'Don't worry, you'll see her again, God will arrange that.' How can that comfort a 6-year-old? Her mummy is *not* coming back to welcome her home from school, to cook her supper, to hug her and tuck her into bed. She is not *ever* coming back. It is traumatic, unbelievable. As a 7-year-old said, 'It's the worstest worst thing.'

Children need clear explanations; they need their own, urgent questions listened to. 'Why did God let Bobby die?' 'I prayed to Jesus to save Daddy, so why didn't he?' Admitting honestly, 'I don't know,' while hugging your child at the same time, is kinder than giving rather elaborate answers you do not fully understand yourself.

For non-believers, these are impossible questions. A 13-year-old dying boy asked his father, 'Will I go to heaven when I die?' His father, an atheist at the time, gave a very honest answer: 'Some people believe this, I'm not sure myself.' *Be honest.* It gets repeated all the time when talking to children, doesn't it? But it is *so* important.

Bringing the church into bereavement

Many families only enter a church for a wedding or a funeral, so when a death occurs, it is not always an automatic signal for a familiar figure from the local church to come and share the family's grief. It is often a stranger who arrives on the doorstep, but the sight of a man in religious dress can give a family confidence. They know he is there to make arrangements for a burial or cremation, and 'having something to do' is helpful to them. A child will trust a priest just as he will (or should) trust a police officer. He will note that his parents respect this man or woman, showing politeness in the same way as they do to his teacher. The priest's presence seems to bring a calming sense of order into a suddenly disordered home.

Clergy can make use of this opportunity to support a family, and happily many do. Thankfully most hold the same views as one clear-thinking parish priest, who told me he never pushes his views onto a family who have not been members of his faith: 'It is not the time.' How right he is: *It is not the time.* Immediately following a fatal tragedy we often hear or see in the media: 'Counsellors have been sent to the bereaved.' Fully trained in comfort and support they may be, but it is often too soon. The parish priest knows that in those bewildering days between the death and the funeral a bereaved family will feel enclosed in an unreal world – for them time is standing still. 'The greatest comfort I can offer is to give great meaning to the well-remembered and worthwhile life of the person who has died.'

Only through this type of contact will any clergy be able to form a relationship of trust with a sorrowing family. Later, in the weeks and months to come, his or her continued presence will be welcome, and talk of their faith listened to. A Sunday school teacher said she also advises all her helpers to wait at least 24 hours before calling on a family after a death. 'When they do call, I tell them it's no good trying to provide easy answers, there aren't any.'

She's right. No church has 'magic' answers to sorrow. No person, no prayers, no faith, can provide the one thing a bereaved child wants – her dead Mummy or Daddy alive again. Religious men or women who acknowledge such helplessness, and admit that even they cannot perform miracles, have a far greater chance of being allowed by that child to provide comforting support.

A Roman Catholic priest voiced similar thoughts with great understanding:

It is not a time for platitudes. It is fundamental to all bereaved persons, and essential to a young child, that the loved person has left them. She needs to be reassured first and foremost that this irreplaceable person truly loved her. That's where I start to console a child. After that, I can help them in their natural and spiritual development. I see my role as not just to arrange and conduct a burial service, but to be available as a friend.

The variety of beliefs among Christians is very wide, and I personally welcome the more ecumenical approach that is growing in pastoral care.

Bereavement counselling in the church

Less than a decade ago, leavers from a Church of England theological college told me they received no formal training in bereavement counselling other than being able to conduct a funeral, and being told to 'visit and take food to the bereaved'. A hospital chaplain admitted that when he began his ministry in the early 1990s he was under the assumption that bereavement did not affect children!

At the same time, the Roman Catholic Church did not offer formal training on bereavement counselling to students during their three-year training, and young priests could be thrown into a parish with no more experience of bereavement in childhood than the loss of a pet cat.

Thankfully, today, bereavement counselling is among the subjects studied during a pastoral year in most theological colleges. Lecturers include doctors and child psychiatrists, social and hospice workers, and counsellors from widows' and parents' circles.

So it is to be hoped that the young clergy of the future will be better equipped than a curate who walked into the home of a newly widowed mother only a few years ago and said, 'I'm afraid I don't know anything about death.'

Funerals

There is a growing trend towards encouraging children of all ages to attend funerals. Widows and widowers, counsellors and child psychiatrists, all stress this as being of vital importance in a family's sharing of grief – and there is plenty of evidence to prove their views. As with all such issues, it must be an individual family's decision – it could be unkind and insensitive to pressure a grieving family either way. Restless toddlers can be distressing to a bereaved parent, and if an older child is very upset at the thought, then he should never be forced to attend.

Neither the surviving parent, nor the children, may be in a fit mental state to take such decisions, but giving children a choice *is* wise, provided they are told beforehand what will happen at the service, where it will take place, and if possible are shown where the grave (if there is to be one) will be.

A Catholic priest was attending, not conducting, a burial service for a family friend's young daughter. At the graveside he felt a small hand slip into his and saw the family's 4-year-old son had been forgotten. At that moment the tiny coffin was lowered into the grave and the little boy began to scream hysterically; the priest had to take him home and comfort him with a warm drink and let him play with his toys – talking could come later. He had been told nothing of what would take place, so that whatever fantasies and fears had been in his little mind must have overwhelmed him at this strange place, and the unmistakable atmosphere of sadness had affected him deeply.

If an understanding minister, or friend, can get the family together a few days before and read through the church or graveside service, choosing hymns and readings together, or planning some well-loved music, it will make it less remote and less dreaded.

One widow, now a counsellor, said she spoke honestly with her children when they said they were afraid of coming to their father's funeral:

> Yes, it will be sad, I'm sure to cry, Dad would understand that. We will have his favourite music and flowers from his garden, and all his friends are coming, and some of yours. The clergyman will talk about Dad. I'd love you to be there, and Aunty will come to sit next to us. But she'll stay at home with you if you feel you'd rather not come.

I love her idea of Aunty sitting with the children. Nothing is sadder than to see children alone at a funeral, their adult relations too grief-stricken to notice them. A well-loved family friend can be allocated to sit near the children – it could be a thoughtful, practical way to help a family. The main point is to see that it is a shared experience, so that no one feels 'left out'. I heard a teenager say how upset and hurt he was that none of the mourners shook *his* hand at his father's funeral – only those of other adults. Happily, today it is not unusual for children to join other family members or friends during the service in saying a few words about their parent or sibling, or perhaps reading out poems they have chosen, or possibly written themselves.

There can, of course, be gross insensitivity from those who ought to know better. A vicar she had never met before walked in on a new widow who had two children aged 9 and 11. 'You won't want them at the funeral, will you?' was his opening remark, and in her state of numbness following the sudden death of her young husband, she agreed with him. Later, she was extremely sad they had not accompanied her – and in time learned that they had felt very left out but had not liked to ask to come.

To compound the hurt, an educational psychologist, who was called in to the younger child six months later for school refusal, started his conversation with the words, 'So you're the boy who didn't go to his father's funeral?'

The service

A girl of 12 and her 15-year-old sister said that the service disappointed them. 'The vicar waffled on a bit about Dad going to heaven, which didn't make up for anything. It's no consolation at the time.' Far more comforting, and of greater warmth to a heartbroken family, is to talk of their loved one's life, to show how cherished it was and how long it will be remembered.

One chaplain said he likes the family to reach the church early:

> I make sure the coffin is there already, with all the family flowers on it – none of this solemn bearing it in which is an added agony. The children realize that the loved Dad or Mum is there with them, they are all together. They can pray or talk among themselves, and then their friends join them and the service starts. It slightly eases the whole occasion. Afterwards, the children walk out *in front of* the coffin – again, it's less sombre, less tense.

I asked another minister if he alters the words of the service according to the children present. 'I choose my words with enormous care,' he said, and I know that care meant compassion. At a student's funeral he addressed the teenage mourners: 'Don't worry if you have doubts about God or feel angry and bitter. Remember we are all here because we loved Charles, so let's share that.'

Secular funerals

Some families believe a religious ceremony would be alien to them; often the deceased has left a request for no church service; others may choose a humanist or interfaith service; even a pagan ceremony can be held – the undertaker will make any arrangements a family wishes. There is always a need for some sort of goodbye, and a short committal service can be comforting. In a crematorium non-hymnal music can be played, or not, as the mourners wish. Sometimes a close friend or relative will say a few words about the person who has died.

Families may find, after the confusion and sorrow of a death, a graveside ceremony is less bewildering for their children than a cremation, and this can also be arranged by the undertaker.

The Humanist Society accepts that death is the natural end of life – that being is synonymous with living. They have no minister to perform a funeral service, but rather an 'officiant'. However, as one officiant said, 'To insist that this life is *all* would be unkind to a family when in grief – it is too dogmatic. After all, it is a bonus to have this life, but they don't want to have a cut-off point.' She encourages bereaved children to celebrate the life of the loved person who has died – and to remember that so much in life is mysterious; we do not know what other worlds exist. Family members, including children, can talk or read out verses at the service.

Green burial grounds are now being provided in many parts of the UK following ever-increasing requests from the public. These peaceful resting places can be less formidable for children. The coffin is often taken there by horse and cart, or on a trolley which the children can help to push. The coffin can be made of wood, though more often it is of wicker, or perhaps cardboard on which young family members can attach drawings or place flowers. The *Natural Death Handbook* (see page 115) gives more details.

Once the funeral is over

The dreaded funeral day, with the agonizing get-together afterwards of unfamiliar relatives, is over. The house is strangely quiet, and the gap in the family is suddenly very noticeable. They would all appreciate someone to talk to, who has time to listen. But any young person will shrink from an aloof stranger who speaks only about his church. One boy of 10 years said, 'He never mentioned Dad once. What did he come for?'

Other clergy show great compassion. A friend told me her two youngsters poured out all sorts of thoughts and worries to a young priest who strolled in and joined in a family game of Monopoly the week after her husband's funeral. 'I'm not good at this game,' he told them. 'I bet your dad was clever at playing it?'

'They were soon asking him to help mend their bikes and give a hand with their homework,' smiled their mother. 'And in time my 11-year-old poured out her confusion over a grave in the ground and a heaven in the sky. She had never done that to me.' This seems to be pastoral care at its best – surely a stronger basis for any future spiritual care than the quasi-theological sayings often brought out as soon as the coffin has been buried.

Many churches are beginning to think on similar lines, though some are short-staffed and incorporate several parishes. Most clergy take upwards of 30 funerals a year – many for families they do not know personally. In large city areas this is inevitable, and only if a church can involve other carers, thus creating small communities for support, will they be able to reach out to distressed families.

If a family belongs to a local church and is included in the close and warm friendship of a young wives' group or prayer circle, or the children are members of a Sunday school, they will find enormous comfort and strength. Such involvement with familiar groups can go a long way to combating the inevitable sense of isolation that bereavement brings. Quakers (the Religious Society of Friends), for example, have no ritual, formal creed or clergy, but the overseer from a local Friends Meeting House can be of great support. Just the presence of another Quaker can bring great comfort to a bereaved family. For a child to be gathered into such a group shows him that people *care*. Tension is eased for the whole family, and death being 'part of life' suddenly makes sense.

Living in a multicultural society

Many of the smaller communities who live away from their roots tend to build up very strong, supportive groups wherever they happen to be. Let's look at some of these minority cultures in Britain:

Buddhism

Buddhism, with its doctrine of brotherhood, encompasses grieving families with strong support. Their children speak of being comforted by the extraordinary calmness with which death is accepted.

Hinduism

Hinduism is one religion that offers a firm social structure, even within the small nuclear families now living in Europe. A strong feature of Hindu attitudes is geared to the acceptance of the inevitable, so that when death occurs it is accepted without anger – death is seen as a door to rebirth. After the death (Hindus are always cremated) there is a ceremony called *Sreda* when food offerings are brought, and the sharing of grief is generous and cathartic. Friends visit the family several times a day for the first week, and relatives stay in the house until the thirteenth day after the death, when the religious ceremonies end.

Islam

When there is a death in a Muslim family, the children are usually told that God gave them life and that same God will take it away when their limited time is up. Devout Muslims discipline themselves to show no emotion at a death lest it should suggest rebellion against God's will. However, it is more common today to display grief openly and children find support during the mourning period (usually one month) when friends visit, bring food, and talk in terms of praise about the person who has died. Meanwhile, only the men (including boys over the age of 12) are allowed to pray in the mosque.

Judaism

The Jewish community provides a bereaved family with outside support by the very nature of their beliefs and rituals. One rabbi describes Judaism as the most 'this life' affirming. Jews believe in an afterlife but give greater consideration to the bereaved who belong to the 'here and now'. 'We don't go in for talking about heaven.'

Following a death, there is an intense seven-day period of mourning within the bereaved home, called a *shiva*. During this time, much food is brought in by relatives and friends, and every night prayers are said together. For the children the visibility of this care, love and support, especially the bringing of food, is very helpful – they realize how much other adults care about their sadness.

Sikhism

Sikhism is essentially a practical community religion, and this is clearly seen when a family is bereaved. Support for the children – financial, social and spiritual – is freely given, without ties or time limits. Believing as they do in reincarnation, few Sikhs regard death as frightening, and children's mourning is helped by this implicit belief. Except in the case of a stillborn child, cremation is always chosen, not burial. This should take place as soon as possible. If in their own country, a funeral pyre would be lit by the eldest son, or the heir to the dead person. In Britain this ritual can be replaced by the pushing of the button at the crematorium.

Having many of these communities living in the UK today should enable us to come closer to tolerating one another's beliefs, and surely a time of death is an opportunity for more than a glimpse into other religions? Where better to start than with the young? As we saw in the previous chapter, all schools are becoming more multicultural, and enable pupils to study and discuss many different beliefs.

Children are naturally very sympathetic and kind – yet they *can* be cruel to others. At a large secondary school in England a Muslim boy was seen crying, for which he was teased and bullied by the rest of his class. But two children asked to visit his home and found that the boy's grandfather had died. His mother, by tradition, was weeping in one room, his father in another. The English children were given food, and made welcome, and the next day they returned to give the mother flowers. The Muslim boy became their friend. They had all learned their first lesson in tolerance and understanding.

I think compassion is probably the word most suited to administer to a sad child. Pity is seldom helpful, and love can be overworked. But compassion means loving with empathy and care, and continues long after formal sympathy has vanished.

Facing alternative answers

There are races and cultures that hold beliefs that are strange to some people – alien or perhaps frightening to others. If children come to you with unusual stories, perhaps of the paranormal, or reincarnation, don't be worried. Do not entirely dismiss their stories either – explain that some cultures believe in them. Remember that bereaved children are now facing a *reality* – death has come into their lives and has actually happened to someone they adore; it's no longer a remote event that happens to other people. Naturally they will be questioning everything they have ever heard or read to do with death and the here-after, and will be ripe to taste the weird offerings of unfamiliar sects. Ouija boards may be tried, the occult considered, but you should encourage them to talk over these things. Don't leave them to face their fears alone.

It is not only young people who seek alternative answers. Hospice workers find some families reluctant to discuss their Christian commitment, yet find those same families secretly visiting faith healers.

A young widow told me how her mother-in-law told her two daughters that she had spoken to her son, their dead father, and that Daddy had sent them a message. 'I only found out when 8-year-old Kitty asked me if she could go to a Spiritualist church to find Daddy. My older daughter was terrified.' If that mother-in-law had discussed her beliefs openly with all the family, before confronting the young girls, it could have enabled them to understand that everyone has their own ways of seeking comfort. Once again, it is worth emphasizing the need for families to talk together.

Where religion is not the answer

Children may question a surviving parent about every aspect of religion. After moving house, one father was desperately trying to comfort his tearful 9-year-old each night. Finally, the little boy told his granny, 'Now we won't see Mummy when she comes back to our old house as a ghost.' Our children's fantasies bring out more emotions than we thought possible.

Religion can sometimes overwhelm parents after a death. One couple whose eldest daughter died thought that they had to deny their natural sadness in order to prove their trust in 'God's purpose'. This unnatural bottling-up of all instinctive sorrow only added to their agony, and their two younger children misinterpreted this behaviour as uncaring.

Grandparents, so supportive in practical ways, sometimes forget that *their* rigid religious belief cannot always help the younger members of the family. Explanations involving a description of God needing the dead parent to work in heaven *may* sometimes offer help to a young adult. But to a small child who wants his father here and now, it can encourage distrust and hatred of the God who has stolen his Daddy.

Far wiser was a college lecturer who I heard talking to his grandchildren:

> In our church it helps us to believe that the part of Mummy we love and remember – her kindness and her love – is not in that dead body in the cemetery ... but in a place where there is no pain, no war, no starving children, no dangers of any kind – just peace and quiet.

Children like to share an adult's thoughts about such an important death. It helps them to feel included, and yet not overwhelmed by dogmatic theories beyond their comprehension.

Explaining death to children

One of the most beautiful explanations of death is contained in the old fable of waterbugs and dragonflies. I've seen adults as well as children moved by the evocative picture it provides.

It uses the analogy of a waterbug's short life underwater for man's short time on earth, and its emergence as a dragonfly as man's life after death. Young children can easily interpret this idea of leaving the old body behind – of never coming back. Doris Stickney has used this in a booklet I would recommend to parents and teachers (see Further reading, page 115).

Teenagers and the church

A church that comforts by offering the possibility of reunion is not always helpful in adolescence. It is like offering a 17-year-old a pension. 'I'd rather have the money now, thanks.' And in the aftermath of tragic death: 'I want Mum here, today, not some vague hope of seeing her when I'm old and dead.'

There is a danger of underestimating the adult thinking of our teenage children. They may appear rebellious and anarchic but many are *very* concerned about moral values; they are beginning to make spiritual searches. We would be wise to take them entirely into our confidence, treat them as equals, confide our doubts: 'Sometimes, illness and suffering make the most faithful Christians wonder if there is a God.'

Melissa, who was inconsolable at her mother's funeral, was baking scones when I visited her family the following month. Covered in flour, she gave me the first smile I had seen since her mother's fatal illness. 'Do you know, I sort of feel Mummy is with me now, she's here all the time. After all, she taught me how to make scones.'

Have you heard a better explanation of 'life everlasting' than that?

9

When a family death
brings relief

We know the sorrow, disruption and despair that follow the death of a family member in a happy home. Think of it in an *un*happy home.

An academic's description of such a situation is 'disordered mourning'. Very apt. Nothing seems to have *any* order. Rejoicing sometimes takes the place of weeping, and grieving is done only for the 'might have been'. Ambivalent emotions abound, and for children all is confusion.

Karen's father had abused her sexually since she was 8 years old, although he was never violent. Then when she was 12 he died. Her relief was enormous, no more fear or shame. But she wept bitterly at his funeral. 'He's still my father. I feel sorry for him.' Another small girl, also sexually abused, expressed her feelings differently. 'I felt like a widow when Dad died.'

The two comments illustrate that it doesn't do to have assumptions when trying to comfort children. The second child had felt her life to be 'living a lie', as though she had been having an illicit affair. Even though she was thankful that she was spared any further deceit, she had never felt conscious of being an 'abused child'. Pathetically adult feelings fought with her childish fear of being 'found out'.

It is not only girls who suffer in this way. Many boys are physically abused by their fathers and older brothers, or emotionally abused by their mothers. Sometimes a whole family lives in fear – perhaps the most stressful of emotions.

Feelings of guilt

Imagine the consequences of a parent's death in such a family. Boys and girls talk of feeling 'bad' and 'worthless'. Years of what felt like punishments have instilled a belief that *they* must be guilty. One little girl thought that if she had been 'better' her dad would not have assaulted her. An older girl said, 'I suppose my mourning took the form of crying for my wrongdoings – I felt dirty. Yet my sister and I danced in our room for joy when that awful man called Dad was dead.'

However awful he was, they are now a fatherless family. The children have a double grief to face: they have to mourn their father, at the same time mourning a father they would love to have had, but never did. They probably always hoped he would turn into their 'dream' daddy. Now he's dead and no amount of wishing can make that happen.

Inevitably, relief creeps in, but it is not really acceptable. Such thoughts are too shameful to mention. Besides, Mum has never believed their stories about Dad anyway. So inside the child is all this bottled-up self-recrimination. If left, it can turn sour, or explode.

Other families are 'abused' by a domineering, nagging mother who 'uses' her children mercilessly, making them her domestic slaves; any pocket money they work for or get from their father she makes them hand over to her. If they refuse, they are beaten, or go without a meal. Fathers seldom believe them when they complain. Such a mother's death can leave children with a suspicious father and a distrust and fear of women.

Loss of fear

There can be very forceful relief at the loss of fear. Graham was the eldest in a boisterous, happy family of five children. At 16 he became involved with a crowd of youngsters who smoked pot – in less than a year he started a life of crime. In spite of strong parental support he was continually put on probation, always sick, always stealing from his mother, soon becoming a heroin addict. He and his friends terrorized the younger children. The big brother they had admired became a terrifying stranger. A week before his nineteenth birthday, Graham died in sordid circumstances. His brothers and sisters knew that now they were safe from his threats. Their tears were of relief, there would be no more ugly scenes and police raiding their home.

But Jenny, the 15-year-old, was unable to join in their relief. At school, her teacher had made her angry. 'He kept saying what a good thing Graham had died and wasn't sick any more, that he would never have been cured.' She kept bursting into tears. 'He was my brother. How dare anyone speak like that. Mum's heartbroken. Why can't people understand?'

Regret and bitterness intrude into all their happy memories – such children truly know the meaning of the word despair. To help them is a long and difficult task. The important thing is to know the family situation. This is where an old friend can be invaluable. It is not enough to know, as Jenny's teacher did, that a father, mother or brother has died. You have to find out the relationships that existed. Even where households appear chaotic, they contain areas of love. Family ties can be very strong even amid anger and violence. Did the children have any affection? Do they know what loving means? Have they ever been hugged or kissed?

For children, death may act as a freezing point: arguments will now never be resolved; apologies will never be offered; a dead parent can never explain his actions; regrets and guilts will be held as though frozen. As the months pass, the thawing-out process may be extremely painful, and many children need very special help – although, incredibly, some children emerge stronger from their experiences.

I've spoken with many counsellors, including those from specific faiths. How would they counsel a child who hated a parent who has just died? They *all* stress that it does no good to ignore that hatred. If you do, the child will end up imprisoned by it. Of course, to get a child to admit this – 'I hated my dad and I'm glad he's dead' – will cause great pain. They may feel that the enormity of their hatred caused the death; after all, they wanted it to happen. To say, 'You didn't *really* hate your daddy, did you, dear?' would confuse an already guilt-ridden child. One counsellor summed up his advice:

> Only if there is someone around whom the child trusts sufficiently, and knows is receptive and caring, will he be able to express his true feelings. Once that happens, a child can be helped to understand that it is not *he* who is guilty, but his parent; then he can learn to forgive that parent, and more importantly, himself for his hatred.

That sounded too much to ask of any young person, let alone one who had suffered abuse, but 14-year-old Harry said that for him it worked. 'Suddenly I was free,' he said. 'I knew it was all in the past. How awful it would be if my dad's problems ruined my whole life.'

Harry is an exceptional young man – able to cope with his future as well as help his mother. But there are still many youngsters who will never be 'free' until someone explains to them: '*You* are not the guilty one.'

To help them understand this, I think that children should be reminded that even in good relationships, where a child has loving parents, there will be some points of regret. 'Why did I say that?' 'Why didn't she do this?' Guilt can creep in and sometimes overshadow regret, upsetting many happy memories. It would surely help children such as Karen and Jenny and Harry to be told this truth, so that they can recognize that they are not alone.

10

How bereavement in childhood affects adult life

When Helga was only 6, her mother died in childbirth, together with the newborn baby, and the little girl was left with a bitter and silent father, who refused to talk about death or dying. Also, he never allowed a mother-figure into their home.

The feeling of abandonment Helga experienced stayed with her for 30 years. After her marriage, she clung to her husband who could not understand the reason for her childlike behaviour; finally he left her. She turned to a clinical psychologist, who understood at once that Helga, now in her forties, was still suffering from her early bereavement. He understood that there was no way to help her until her childhood sadness was recognized and attended to. He said, 'She will always have a scar – but hopefully the right therapy will prevent it putrefying, as it were, the rest of her emotional body.'

The relationship that the psychologist was able to find with Helga was life-saving. He not only discovered the cause of Helga's depression, but pointed it out to her, showing her that it was up to her to 'leap over it'. It was to be a painful process – but that is what bereavement counselling is all about, giving people a helping hand over these hurdles that have been avoided in the past, so they can carry on with their lives.

Many studies now link adult psychiatric disorders with the death of a parent in childhood. Details of such studies vary, though all believe age to be a significant factor. A child under 10 when a parent dies is at high risk for future problems, and girls who lose their mothers under the age of 12 can be prone to depressive illness.

However, dogmatic statements and statistics can be misleading, and leading psychiatrists acknowledge that 'even the evidence of a high number of adults receiving psychiatric treatment having been bereaved in childhood is not convincing'. Pathological grieving can be due to many contributing factors – both before and after the actual parental death. Death creates instability in a family, and this alone can lead to great insecurity and loss of purpose in young people, leaving them vulnerable and likely to collapse in the face of problems as they grow up.

In favourable circumstances – and even in fairly disordered ones – most children do cope successfully with the death of a parent or sibling. Psychiatrists are the first to admit they never meet this silent majority. Professional research naturally deals with those children who were *not* able to survive the stress of bereavement, and often includes patients who were already in therapy at the time of the study. Most bereaved children grow into well-balanced, sensitive and caring adults, able to face life and its many setbacks. They carry the scars of their bereavements, but are not disabled by them.

It is easy to lay blame for mental disorders or behavioural problems onto childhood bereavement – but this is often 'making excuses' for what may be either family or social problems. Two child psychiatrists I spoke with said that in their experience childhood bereavement plays a causal role in only a small minority of mental illness cases.

Lingering grief

However, I feel strongly that the grief that lingers into adult life *is* in part also due to the death, regardless of how that loss is handled. Love of a parent is the first love a child knows, and for the average child the death of a mother or father will be a gigantic loss, overwhelming in its impact. Naturally much will depend on how the parent responded to and nurtured that love, as well as how the loss was handled.

Whether or not the feelings they suffer – withdrawal, anger, disruptive behaviour – later turn into a pathological problem depends on several factors: the circumstances of the death, the relationships that existed between the child and the person who has died, and the support the bereaved child receives.

Happily, strong childhood emotions can, and frequently do, result in potential growth from loss. Mary is approaching middle age now, but remembers the day her father died when she was 10. 'I felt as if a huge oak tree had fallen down ... But I am a living branch of that dead tree.' She was one of the lucky children. She had a supportive, encouraging family, who never let the children be uprooted with that tree, or crushed by its fall.

Pathological forms of grief

Withdrawal or delayed mourning, chronic or distorted grief, are most likely to occur in the more unusual cases, perhaps after a suicide, or if a child has witnessed a violent murder, or even within an unloving family, or outside any community support.

Children who have the most severe grief reactions, which persist into adulthood, are nearly always those who had no support in their early bereavement, and were given no opportunity to mourn. The surviving parent was too distressed or too ignorant to be of any help, and no professional or neighbour was ever alerted.

I also feel great sadness for those who suffer lifelong consequences of a childhood bereavement simply because the adults around them at the time were unable to face the reality of death. Gladys, even when in her sixties, had a distrust of all adults, and has led a lonely life. She was only 7 years old when her father 'went away'. At first, she was told he would be home 'soon', but then it was always 'next year' and if she pressed for details, she was told to stop fussing. She told school friends her father was abroad. When she was 20, her mother died, and only then did she find out from the family lawyer that her father had been dead since she was 7.

Gladys cries easily even now. 'It is as if I'm making up for those years when I should have been mourning.'

Professional or non-professional help?

I am not among those who advise avoiding psychiatrists at all costs. Indeed I am particularly grateful for their help and encouragement to me in writing this book. I have to say, however, that this is one area in which the old cliché about a little knowledge being a dangerous thing is very apt. To read or listen to the professionals discussing death in their 'bereavement language' could and sadly does at times alienate a person wishing to find help for someone they know to be seriously disturbed.

For a newly bereaved child, the ideal help will come from a close family member or friend who can provide love, security and a listening heart. In a child who appeared to survive the initial crisis well, but who in reality was hiding searing grief, signs of a disturbed personality development may appear a year or more later, perhaps during adolescence or beyond. A teenage girl may become pregnant through a desire to have someone of her own to love, or be abnormally overwhelmed by a broken love affair. Such isolated incidents seldom require more than the support of close friends. It is when the original loss remains an unconquerable emotional burden or stress that cannot be coped with that help is needed.

There are now many support groups who give compassionate counselling to such young people, who may well be enabled to release their pent-up emotions, survive their depression, and learn to control their lives.

But if none of these help lines have been available during the years following bereavement, depressive symptoms in adulthood will suggest that deep emotional wounds have never healed. A psychotherapist or experienced counsellor can usually, at this stage, provide the 'reflective talk' and supporting advice that is desperately needed. Occasionally a person can be so deeply 'imprisoned' in their depressed state that they will need further medical help. The work of professionals in psychiatric treatment can be as life-saving as that of doctors and surgeons.

Sadly, it is not always those in the greatest need who seek and find such help. 'You'll never get me to a shrink!' is a familiar cry; while for others ignorance, lack of money or family opposition stand in their way. Some, like Gladys, waste a lifetime in isolated sorrow.

How can we help?

How can we, whether we are trained counsellors, teachers, clergy, medical staff, parents, grandparents, friends or relatives, prevent a bereaved child from suffering mental disorders in her adult life?

To be there, and *to be honest* – that is a good start. The bereaved suffer insensitivity from all sides – from ignorant friends, impatient doctors and teachers, and from over-professional or arrogant experts. But a kindly uncle, sensitive teacher or friendly neighbour can act as a refuge in their time of chaos.

Children who have experienced horrendous events, witnessed violence and death, been abused and neglected, often need psychiatric help in coping with such disasters while they are still young; but children who have been 'protected' from the knowledge of such disasters have suffered *more* in later life when they discover the truth. Not being told the truth can be more frightening than the truth itself.

One of the few good things to come from a tragedy is that those who have been through the experience make the best helpers for others. However, you will remember, if you have been through such a time yourself, that what you did *not* want was to hear an account of someone else's tragedy; you needed a good listener, someone who cared about *you*.

Despite the growing awareness that children *do* suffer grief, *do* need time to mourn, attitudes are slow to change. 'Don't let's talk about death, it's over, let's get back to normal,' still tends to dominate advice to the bereaved. If being 'brave' means 'don't cry', then this admonition to a child is too cruel to contemplate. If a child – if anyone – cannot cry when their parent dies, what sort of society have we created? No wonder psychiatric treatment is increasingly needed as we become more and more 'civilized'.

But hopefully we are leaving behind the reactionary period when death was unmentionable, especially in front of the children. In Britain now, as earlier chapters show, there are counselling groups, self-help circles, seminars, lectures and guidelines for all professionals who come in contact with bereaved children. Hospital and hospice care extends well beyond the bedside, and professional research is gradually being put to good use in practical ways – helping the parents and carers of bereaved children.

Jonathan, now a middle-aged father, is deeply grateful for our new awareness of children and their feelings. Recently a hospice nurse remarked to him, 'We recognize here that bereaved siblings do have feelings.' To her amazement, he broke down and cried.

> When I was 15 my teenage sister died. My father had left home and all my relatives kept telling me I had to support my mother. No one ever recognized I was grieving too. After all these years, it is very comforting to talk with someone who understands.

To talk with someone who understands. That is basically all a bereaved child is seeking. If you can talk, and listen – really listen, with your heart – you may well prevent another sad little girl or boy from wrapping themselves up in their grief until they become enclosed in an isolated world from which a very disturbed adult will emerge.